CANCER
DECONSTRUCTED

*The real causes of cancer and how to reverse it
with energy medicine and natural remedies*

DR. GERALD H. SMITH

Digitally produced in the United States of America

Cancer Deconstructed
- *Real causes of cancer*
- *How the AMA, FDA, and Big Pharma suppresed the real cures*
- *How to reverse cancer with natural remedies and integrative medicine*

Author: **Dr. Gerald H. Smith**

Editing by: **Dr. Gerald H. Smith**

Front cover design: **Johanna Bellerose**

All case photographs taken by: **Dr. Gerald H. Smith**

Main category: **Health**

First Edition release date: September 18, 2020

Publisher: **International Center For Nutritional Research, Inc.**

303 Corporate Drive East • Langhorne, PA 19047

Conversion/Production: **The Gombach Group**

Web site: **www.icnr.com and www.ghsdoc.com**

TABLE OF CONTENTS

    a. The contribution of cytotoxic chemotherapy to 5-year survival in adult malignancies.

    b. Chemotherapy spreading cancer

    c. Chemotherapy may make breast cancer more aggressive and likely to spread

    d. It's been known for years that chemotherapy can trigger tumor growth

    e. Conventional oncologists aren't likely to explain the many options for treatment

    a. Access to natural cure's research blocked by AMA

    b. Alternative cancer therapy suppression

    c. FDA, American Medical Association, and Big Pharma Suppression of natural cancer therapies that work

    d. Rife frequency generator

    e. Antineoplastons: another suppressed breakthrough against cancer

    f. FDA approval of antineoplastons

    g. Connecting the dots

    h. Hitler's gift to the world - The cure for cancer

PREFACE

ancer Deconstructed was written to expose the fraud in the cancer industry. The pharmaceutical cartel, American Medical Association, the FDA, and the media have created an illusion that there are over 100 different types of cancer and that they have done extensive research and meticulously developed special cancer treatment protocols for each type of cancer. This industry has spent billions of dollars brainwashing physicians and the public to buy into this lie. If the cancer industry's treatments are so miraculous and work so well, why do they constantly have to suppress real breakthrough technologies and eliminate any physician who has developed treatments that are noninvasive, less expensive, less side effects, and have well documented proof of success. The answer is simple. They do not have the answers, they are generating well over 450 billion dollars a year in revenue, and lastly they are afraid of the competition that can destroy their golden goose. Most oncologists make more money from their kickbacks from the pharmaceutical companies; they could donate their medical salaries to charity and still have plenty of money in the bank.

After reading the science backed information presented, your cancer bubble will be broken. For most readers, it will be a major shock. The information presented was partially based on my own personal experiences dealing with my wife's breast cancer and stage III ovarian cancer. I saw first-hand how this industry utilizes fear tactics to intimidate their victims. Once you become familiar with what cancer really is about, the fear will quickly dissipate and you will have a totally different perspective on cancer and the integrative technologies that are available to reverse it. I invite you to participate on an exciting journey along the road less travelled to learn the truth about cancer.

BIOGRAPHY

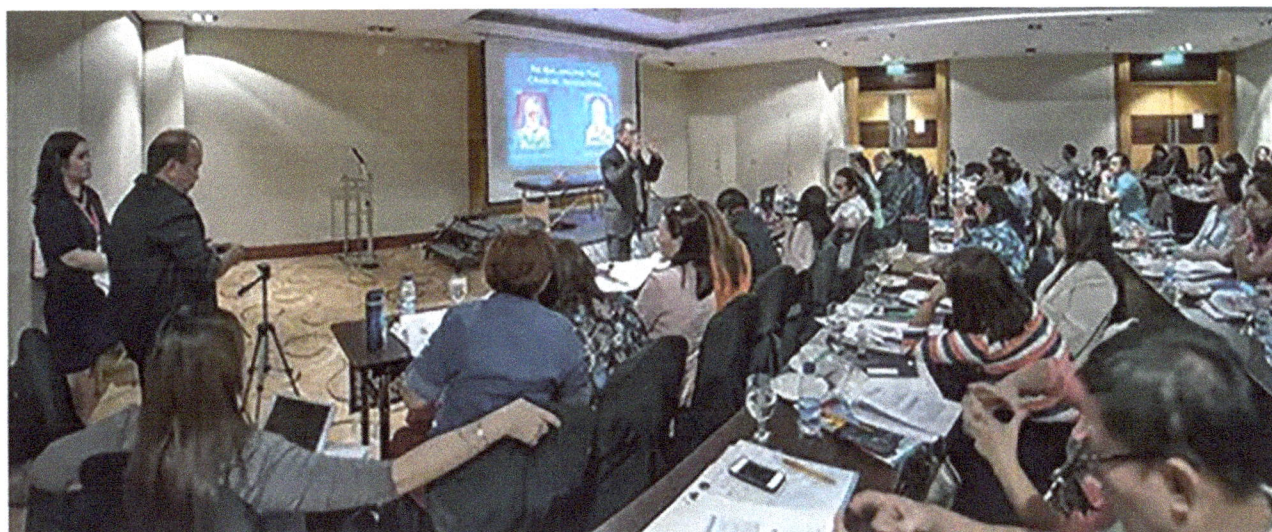

Doctor Smith Presenting A Lecture in Manila

Doctor Smith graduated Temple School of Dentistry in 1969 and completed a two-year tour of active duty as a captain in the U.S. Army Dental Corp. After practicing conventional dentistry for four years, Dr. Smith completed a two-year post-graduate orthodontic program in 1976. Sir, Doctor Smith is a Knight Hospitaller a dedicated professional organization dating back to the year 1050. The Knights Hospitallers have official recognition from the United Nations and the Pope for their tremendous humanitarian work with the poor. Doctor Smith is certified by the World Organization For Natural Medicine to practice natural medicine.

Dr. Smith's broad base of post-graduate training has enabled him to integrate many health care specialties. He has accumulated an impressive list of credentials, which includes lecturing at Walter Reed Army Medical Center, National Academy of General Dentistry, Academy of Head, Neck and Facial Pain, Yonsei Memorial Hospital in Seoul Korea and dozens of guest lecture appearances at national and international symposia. He holds membership in the World Organization For Natural Medicine. He has been an active member of the Holistic Dental Association since 1993, past-president of the Holistic Dental Association and editor of their professional journal from 2003 to 2006. He also served as past-president of the Pennsylvania Craniomandibular Society.

Dr. Smith is a recognized international authority and pioneer in craniomandibular somatic disorders with a focus on resolving chronic pain. Dr. Smith was the first researcher in the world to document cranial bone motion by means of his ground breaking research and development of the Dental Orthogonal Radiographic Analysis System. He was also the first researcher in the world to discover how to resolve chronic pain by removing tension patterns within the human skull by means of the Occlusal Cranial Balancing Technique. He is author of two landmark textbooks for professionals, *Cranial-Dental-Sacral Complex* and *Dental Orthogonal Radiographic Analysis*. He has also written important books for the lay person, *Headaches Aren't Forever* and *Reversing Cancer: A Journey From Cancer to Cure* — a survivors guide for understanding the nature of cancer, restoring the immune system, psychological healing, destroying cancer, and regeneration. He has also published several downloadable E-books, *Alternative Treatments For Conquering Chronic Pain, Remove the "Splinters" and Watch the Body Heal,* and his latest book *Cancer Deconstructed*. Doctor Smith's fifty years of clinical research has identified several of the major missing links for successfully treating dentally related medical issues, cancer, and chronic pain.

In addition, Dr. Smith has published over thirty articles and contributed chapters to several professional books, developer of the Physiologic Adaptive Range Concept, Occlusal Cranial Balancing Technique, Quantum Testing Technique and a special dental x-ray analysis system for measuring cranial bone motion. He holds two US Patents: a unique precision attachment for dental fixed bridgework and second patent for a flash adaptor to facilitate taking intraoral photographs. Doctor Smith is also president of the International Center For Nutritional Research, Inc. and he still maintains a private practice in Bucks County Pennsylvania, where he focuses his integrative healing concepts on chronic pain patients.

CANCER DECONSTRUCTED

INTRODUCTION

From my fifty plus years of clinical practice, I would have to state that one of the most frightening emotional traumas a person can face is receiving a diagnosis of cancer. I attribute this to the simple fact that people have been conditioned to fear cancer. In reality, cancer is a survival mechanism that the body employs to stay alive. When the cells are deprived of oxygen, the innate intelligence of the cell modifies its software allowing it to convert glucose into energy via a fermentation process (like in the production of wine or beer). In 1931, Dr. Otto Warburg won the Nobel Prize in Physiology for this discovery. Why has his research been ignored for so many years? The answer is simple. Cancer treatment in the United States generates over 450 billion dollars in revenue. Follow the money.

Cancer Deconstructed was written for the layperson to understand the nature of cancer, noninvasive treatments, and to remove the fear factor. Ignorance breeds fear. There is an inverse ratio in which the less one knows about cancer the more fear the word generates. The information provided is designed to dispel many of the myths that surround cancer. An astute philosopher once stated, "I would rather walk alone than with the crowd going in the wrong direction." Review of the medical literature documents that conventional cancer treatment has a 2.3% success rate in the US. Once one understands that conventional medicine's treatment goals are to kill the cancer with toxic chemicals (chemotherapy), invasive therapies like radiation and surgery, while paying little or no attention to the real cause, which is hypoxia and a toxic terrain.

The physiology of all cancers is the same. It makes no difference if its brain cancer, prostate cancer, or breast cancer, the causative factor is an oxygen deficiency and toxic terrain. When the oxygen level drops below thirty-five percent, cancer forms as a survival mechanism. When medicine tells the public that there is specific chemotherapy drugs for the 100 plus types of cancer, they are verifying that they do not understand the nature of cancer. As a cancer patient, you better do your homework so you can make a more informed decision regarding your treatment. Sometimes an integrated approach using the best technologies of conventional and natural medicine may prove to be the best avenue. The key is if you do not investigate the options you will never know what's available. Remember your LIFE depends upon it.

PRELUDE

MEDICINE IN THE TWENTY-FIRST CENTURY

The New Millennium has ushered in a major paradigm shift in medicine. The seeds have started to germinate and practitioners are slowly starting to look for and treat the underlying cause(s). Based on concepts of quantum physics and an integration of many specialities this unique paradigm is called Energy Medicine. Based on intelligent evolution, previous research, patented technologies, and outside the box innovative thinking a more comprehensive evaluation and treatment approach now exists. Embracing this knowledge the enlightened practitioner has the ability to look at the patient globally and incorporate factors which traditional medicine reject, discount or are not even aware.

Because the true nature of cancer has been suppressed by the FDA, AMA, pharmaceutical cartel, and the conventional media, physicians and the public have been kept ignorant by design. Suppression comes in many forms: character assassination of the researchers; false narratives regarding the remedies; published disinformation to frighten the public, research centers being burned down; FTC law suits claiming mislabeling; and even researchers being "suicided."

In order to understand the nature of cancer, a tapestry must be created of discoveries from many fields of science and woven into a recognizable landscape. Once one reviews the research of Dr. Otto Warburg, Nobel Prize Winner in Physiology for discovering the physiologic cause of cancer, and Dr. William F. Koch's discovery of the three factors in the production of cancer, and Dr. Fritz Albert Popp's discovery of biophotons and the characteristic of carcinogens blocking DNA repair you will quickly realize that the cancer establishment has been blatantly lying about cancer for over 100 years. The information presented is a rude awakening but also exhilarating because now we have answers to reverse cancer with natural remedies and noninvasive modalities.

CHAPTER 1

CONVENTIONAL CANCER TREATMENT HOAX

The internationally known medical researcher, lecturer, author, and clinical practitioner, William F. Koch, MD, PhD, stated, "Philosophy does not retain the notion that nature is self-destructive, for if it were self-destructive, it has had in the ages that have passed plenty of chance to cease to exist. Therefore, we cannot hold the view that cancer has accidentally or purposely come into existence to destroy the body that produces it, nor that it is the great blunder of nature, as the pathologist would claim."

Cancer like most other "diseases" has been politicized and monetized. On December 23, 1971, President Nixon followed through on his promise as he signed the National Cancer Act into law. Since that declaration of the "War on Cancer," medicine is no closer to a cure than in 1971. The reason is obvious to anyone who understands how cells function. Conventional medicine focuses their efforts on killing the cancer rather than seeking out the underlying causes: hypoxia (low oxygen), corrupted cell membranes, low cell membrane potential, and a toxic terrain. My prediction is that conventional medicine will never wake up because they have the best academic welfare system going. Why kill the golden goose and all the financial research grants.

The cause of cancer was known back in the early 1930's as well as the cure, and this gift to humanity has been suppressed by the FDA, AMA, and pharmaceutical cartel for all these years. In 1934 under the guidance of Dr. Arthur Kendall, then president of Northwestern Medical School, Dr. E.C. Rosenow, then head of bacteriology at the Mayo Clinic, and Dr.

Milbank Johnson, then president of the Southern California Medical Society they conducted a study. The group was given sixteen terminally ill cancer patients. These cancer patients were all treated with Royal Raymond Rife's frequency generator. In one hundred and thirty days, all the cancer patients were cured. That's when it all hit the fan. In one year, eleven research centers in the US that were testing Dr. Rife's frequency technology mysteriously burned down. The FDA visited physician's offices and confiscated their Rife generators. Dr. Rosenow, never used or spoke about the Rife Technology ever again. Dr. Arthur Kendall disappeared and was later located living on a 300 acre farm in Mexico. Dr. Milbank Johnson mysteriously died the night before he was to give a press conference regarding the success of Dr. Rife's cure for cancer. When Dr. Johnson's body was exhumed six months later, it was discovered that there was arsenic in his toothpaste. Another testament to the fact that the establishment does not want any cancer cures or competition.

The FDA, American Medical Association, and the big pharmaceutical companies effectively use mind control techniques to combat any clinically proven cancer therapy. Their first line of assault focuses on character assassination of the scientist who made the discovery. Articles start appearing in professional journals dismissing the efficacy of the treatment and they will even go as far as calling it quackery to further frighten physicians and the public. The controlled media then starts their campaign that this treatment may be harmful and of course you should talk to your doctor about it before using it. When these tactics fail, they employ their high priced attorneys to get the Federal Trade Commission to take action for faulty labeling. If they do not succeed they will initiate a barrage of grand jury investigations until they find the best judge money can buy to get the verdict they want.

If your oncologist recommends chemotherapy for your cancer treatment, think again. The following medical literature review will burst both your oncologist's and your bubble.

The Contribution of Cytotoxic Chemotherapy to 5-year Survival in Adult Malignancies.

Three Australian medical doctors did a literature search, for randomized clinical trials reporting a 5-year survival benefit attributable solely to cytotoxic chemotherapy in adult malignancies.

The total number of newly diagnosed cancer patients for 22 major adult malignancies was determined from cancer registry data in Australia and from the Surveillance Epidemiology and End Results data in the USA for 1998. For each malignancy, the absolute number to benefit was the product of (a) the total number of persons with that malignancy; (b) the proportion or subgroup(s) of that malignancy showing a benefit; and (c) the percentage increase in 5-year survival due solely to cytotoxic chemotherapy. The overall contribution was the sum total of the absolute numbers showing a 5-year survival benefit expressed as a percentage of the total number for the 22 malignancies.

Results

The overall contribution of curative and adjuvant cytotoxic chemotherapy to 5-year survival in adults was estimated to be 2.3% in Australia and 2.1% in the USA.

Conclusion

As the 5-year relative survival rate for cancer in Australia is now over 60%, it is clear that cytotoxic chemotherapy only makes a minor contribution to cancer survival. To justify the continued funding and availability of drugs used in cytotoxic chemotherapy, a rigorous evaluation of the cost-effectiveness and impact on quality of life is urgently required.

Chemotherapy Spreading Cancer

Dr. Lee Cowden says most people don't die from their cancer; they die from the side effects of treatment. While the "war against cancer" is moving toward more personalized and so-called "precision medicine" treatments, the old standby model of "cut, poison and burn," via surgery, chemotherapy and radiation, is still widely used and regarded as the standard of care for many cancer cases. This paradigm is barbaric by any standard especially in light of proven noninvasive therapies that are kinder to the body and preserve the patient's quality of life.

One of the major problems with chemotherapy is its indiscriminate toxicity, which poisons your body systemically in an attempt to kill cancer cells. There have long been signs that this model has fatal flaws and may cause more harm than good. In the case of the breast cancer chemotherapy drug Tamoxifen, patients must trade one risk for another, as while it may reduce breast cancer, it more than doubles women's risk of uterine cancer.

Serious, sometimes-fatal side effects of chemotherapy are common (acute myeloid leukemia, heart attack, permanent damage to your heart, lungs, chemo brain [cognitive impairment due to destruction of neurons], nerve endings, kidneys, suppression of the immune system, or reproductive organs). As mentioned above, serious unforeseen effects that spread the cancer will make your cancer prognosis worse instead of better. The more common transient side effects may include: brain fog, nausea, hair loss, fatigue, depression, sense of not feeling well, insomnia, and a loss of appetite. This loss of quality of life is rarely mentioned by the oncologists.

Writing in the journal Science Translational Medicine, researchers from the Albert Einstein College of Medicine revealed that giving chemotherapy prior to surgery for breast cancer may promote disease metastasis, or the growth and spread of cancer to other areas of the body. This, in turn, greatly increases a woman's risk of dying from the disease.

Chemotherapy May Make Breast Cancer More Aggressive and Likely to Spread

Preoperative chemotherapy, known as neoadjuvant chemotherapy, is often offered to women because it may help shrink tumors, which increases the likelihood that women will receive lumpectomy surgery instead of a full mastectomy. After performing tests on mice and human tissue, however, the researchers found that doing so may increase the likelihood of metastasis by increasing what are known as "tumor microenvironments of metastasis." These are sites on blood vessels that special immune cells flock to. If the immune cells hook up with a tumor cell, they usher it into a blood vessel like a Lyft picking up a passenger. Since blood vessels are the highways to distant organs, the result is metastasis, or the spread of cancer to far-flung sites."

When mice with breast cancer or given human breast tumors were given the chemotherapy, it altered the tumor microenvironment in ways that made them more conducive to cancer spread, including:

- Increasing the number of immune cells that transport cancer cells into blood vessels
- Making blood vessels more permeable to cancer cells
- Making tumor cells more mobile

In mice, chemotherapy treatment doubled the number of cancer cells in the bloodstream and lungs compared to mice that did not receive the treatment. Further, in 20 human patients who received common chemotherapy drugs, the tumor microenvironments also became more favorable to cancer spread. As The Telegraph noted:

"It is thought the toxic medication switches on a repair mechanism in the body which ultimately allows tumors to grow back stronger. It also increases the number of 'doorways' on blood vessels which allow cancer to spread throughout the body."

Further, researchers wrote in a 2012 Journal of Clinical Oncology editorial, "Unfortunately, neoadjuvant chemotherapy does not seem to improve overall survival, as demonstrated in the National Surgical Adjuvant Breast and Bowel Project (NSABP) B18 trial, among others." This means women may be trading a potential increased risk of cancer metastasis for a treatment that doesn't even improve their chances of survival.

It's Been Known for Years That Chemotherapy Can Trigger Tumor Growth

While the news that chemotherapy may encourage cancer spread may sound surprising, it's not a new discovery. In 2012, researchers found chemotherapy for prostate cancer caused DNA damage in healthy cells and caused them to secrete more of a protein called WNT16B, which boosts tumor growth and may encourage cancer cells to develop resistance to treatment.

"WNT16B, when secreted, would interact with nearby tumor cells and cause them to grow, invade and, importantly, resist subsequent therapy," study co-author Dr. Peter Nelson, of the Fred Hutchinson Cancer Research Center.

In the journal Nature Medicine, the researchers further noted, "The expression of WNT16B in the prostate tumor microenvironment attenuated the effects of cytotoxic chemotherapy in vivo, promoting tumor cell survival and disease progression" and "… Damage responses in benign cells … may directly contribute to enhanced tumor growth kinetics."

While research continues to reveal that chemotherapy's effects are wide-reaching and devastating to healthy cells, it's also been shown — at least as far back as 2004 — that "chemotherapy only makes a minor contribution to cancer survival."

Separate research revealed that out of nearly 2,000 patients receiving chemotherapy, 161 deaths occurred within 30 days of the treatment. Nearly 8 percent of them were classified as related to the chemotherapy (and another nearly 16 percent were unclassified due to insufficient information).

Further, as mentioned, chemotherapy can increase the risk of subsequent cancer, such as therapy-related acute myeloid leukemia (tAML), "a rare but highly fatal complication of cytotoxic chemotherapy." Researchers noted that tAML cases occur nearly five times more often in adults treated with chemotherapy than they do in the general population.

Conventional Oncologists Aren't Likely to Explain the Many Options for Treatment

Upon receiving a cancer diagnosis, many people assume their only options for treatment are chemotherapy, surgery or radiation. Only you and your health care team can make the decision on how to best pursue treatment, but you should know that conventional providers are unlikely to think outside the box or tell you about alternative treatments.

Oncology is the only specialty in medicine that is allowed and even encouraged to sell drugs at massive profits — typically in excess of 50 percent — and cancer drugs are, as a general category, the most expensive medications in all of medicine to begin with. Oncologists actually get commissions, which can be as much as two million dollars, for the chemotherapy drugs they sell, and with that type of incentive, it's nearly impossible to imagine them actively offering alternatives.

Oncologists are further constrained by the "standard of care" prescribed by oncology medical boards and the drug industry. If they go against the established standard of care, they're susceptible to having their license reprimanded or even taken away. As a result, patients are typically forced to go it alone if they don't want to go the conventional route, which is unfortunate because there are many promising alternative treatments.

A shocking admission by the editor of the world's most respected medical journal, The Lancet, is saying that medical research is UNRELIABLE AT BEST IF NOT COMPLETELY FRAUDULENT! Lancet editor, Richard Horton "… states bluntly that major pharmaceutical companies falsify or manipulate tests on the health, safety, and effectiveness of their various drugs by taking samples too small to be statistically meaningful or hiring test labs or scientists where the lab or scientist has blatant conflicts of interest such as pleasing the drug company to get further grants." In reality, what the conventional medical model for cancer and other medical illnesses offer is a pure illusion.

The medical cartel has no vested interest to get you well. It's more profitable to foster a cash cow dependent on daily intake of medications and expensive chemotherapy drugs. The history of medicine has always been to suppress the truth and kill the messenger and there is a long list of dead physicians who discovered major cures for cancer.

> *"You can fool all the people some of the time, and some of the people all the time, but you cannot fool all the people all the time."* Abraham Lincoln

CHAPTER 2

CANCER REMEDIES SUPPRESSED

Access to Natural Cure's Research Blocked by AMA

In the 1930's, the pharmaceutical industry orchestrated the placement of Dr. Morris Fishbein as president of the American Medical Association. One of his jobs was to prevent the listing of any research dealing with natural remedies from being listed in the index medicus. In other words, anyone who tried to locate this type of research would not be able to find it listed in the medical literature.

Alternative Cancer Therapy Suppression

For anyone interested in learning more about how the FDA, American Medical Association, and the pharmaceutical industry suppressed major natural cancer therapy breakthroughs, I urge them to read an incredible investigative book written by Daniel Haley called *Politics in Healing*. Haley exquisitely documents 12 medical researcher's stories to support his theory that the AMA, FDA, and big pharmaceutical companies conspire to prevent new ideas from entering medical research and practice. His subjects include Andrew Ivy, who advocated the discredited anticancer drug Krebiozen; anticancer herbalist Harry Hoxsey; anticancer blood researcher Gaston Naessens; and antineoplastin researcher Stanislaw Burzynski. Those persecuted medical investigators are fairly well known, but some of Haley's other cases concern forgotten men like William F. Koch, developer of the antipolio drug Glyoxylide, whom many may find more interesting because of their obscurity. The stories of all 12 are often absent from current medical histories, which alone makes this book worthwhile. Haley presents an in-depth coverage of their suppression; after reading the well documented facts of these researchers who were victims of organized medicine, you can make up your own opinion as to the unscrupulous tactics used to suppress their discoveries.

FDA, American Medical Association, and Big Pharma Suppression of Natural Cancer Therapies that Work

The medical cartel utilizes a planned approach to neutralize any alternative approach that presents competition to their patented drugs. Their first wave of attacks usually comes in the form of tagging the alternative breakthrough technology as unscientific, quackery, and dangerous. Then they proceed to character assassinate the scientist, prevent his research from being published, and if published force the journal to retract the research articles. They then arrange articles written by their quack doctors in "prestigious" medical journals claiming that the remedies do not work, the research is flawed, and that physicians should not use it. They will even go the extent of using deception to lure the researcher into a study, sabotage it, and then have the Federal Trade Commission charge them with mislabeling. When these tactics fail, they go into high gear. Their high priced legal department starts law suits, grand jury investigations, and even getting the Federal Trade Commission to file charges. Their primary objective is to bankrupt the researcher by piling up legal fees and ultimately get governmental agencies to ban their therapy based on bogus allegations. Remember Big Pharma owns the best judges money can buy.

Rife Frequency Generator

It's hard to believe, that the "War on Cancer" was won back in the 1920s and 1930s, but the results were suppressed from the world. Royal Raymond Rife successfully isolated the filterable cancer virus in 1932 and repeated his procedure 104 consecutive times with identical results! Rife proved that the BX cancer virus had four distinct forms and that any one of these forms can change into BX cancer within 36 hours when the medium on which it was growing was altered; he also was able to replicate this conversion 300 times with identical results. Rife said, "In reality, it is not the bacteria themselves that produce the disease, but the chemical constituents of these microorganisms enacting upon the unbalanced cell metabolism of the human body that in actuality produce the disease. He also believed, if the metabolism of the human body is perfectly balanced or poised, it is susceptible to NO disease."

Rife invented a special light microscope with a prism and a unique light source that enabled him to discover the mortal oscillatory frequency that could kill bacteria, viruses, mold, fungi, yeast, and cancer cells; his research uncovered the fact that every organism vibrates at a signature frequency. He also theorized and proved that subjecting the cancer virus or any other microorganism to its mortal oscillatory frequency at which it vibrated, would literally explode the disease-causing organism without damaging the surrounding tissues. Rife successfully utilized his technology on isolated viruses and then successfully treated over 400 animals with tumors.

In 1934, a special medical study was conducted at the University of Southern California. The research team was headed by Dr. Arthur Kendall, dean of Northwestern Medical School in Chicago, Dr. Edward C. Rosenow, head bacteriologist from the Mayo Clinic, Dr. Milbank Johnson, then president of the Southern California Medical Association, and five other prestigious researchers. These highly qualified scientists were given 16 terminally ill cancer patients to be treated with Rife's Frequency Generator. After treatment for 130 days, all sixteen cancer patients were cured. Of interest was the fact that in one year eleven research centers in the US that were validating Rife's technology mysteriously burn down. Following the successful study, it all hit the fan. Dr. Kendall disappeared and retreated to a 300 acre farm in Mexico; Dr. E.C. Rosenow stopped using Rife's equipment and stopped talking about the technology; Dr. Johnson mysteriously died the night before he was to give a press conference on the successful cure of the sixteen terminally ill cancer patients. Six months after his death his body was exhumed and they found cyanide in his toothpaste. Why then have we NOT heard about this great discovery? The answer is simple. Cancer therapy generates over 450 billion dollars a year in revenue. In addition, oncologists are the only physicians that get kick backs from the big pharmaceutical companies on the chemo drugs they push. If you have a golden goose, why would you want to kill it?

Antineoplastons: Another Suppressed Breakthrough Against Cancer

Dr. Stanislaw Burzynski, a nationally and internationally recognized physician/investigator, pioneered the use of biologically active peptides for the treatment of cancer. In 1967, at the age of 24, Dr. Burzynski graduated first in his class of 250 students from the Medical Academy in Lublin, Poland. It was at this time that he identified naturally occurring human peptides, which were deficient in cancer patients. He concluded that these peptides played a role in preventing the growth of cancer cells. In 1968, he earned a PhD degree and became one of the youngest physician/investigators in Poland to hold both a MD and PhD degrees.

Between 1970 and 1977, he received funding from the National Cancer Institute (NCI) for his work as a Principal investigator and Assistant Professor at the Baylor College of Medicine in Houston, TX. During this time he authored/coauthored numerous publications, including those detailing his work on naturally occurring human peptides and their effect on cancer – some of which were co-authored by investigators associated with the M.D. Anderson Cancer Center or the Baylor College School of Medicine. In May 1977, Dr. Burzynski received a Certificate of Appreciation from the Baylor College of Medicine that acknowledged his contributions to the 'Advancement of Medical Education, Research, and Health Care'.

In 1977 the Burzynski Clinic was established in Houston, TX. Since then, more than 10,000 patients have received treatment at the clinic, including more than 2,300 cancer patients who have been treated in FDA reviewed and Institutional Review Board (IRB) approved clinical trials program of Antineoplastons, investigational agents that derived from Dr. Burzynski's early investigations of naturally occurring human peptides. Currently, new FDA-reviewed Phase II and III clinical studies utilizing Antineoplastons are awaiting funding approval prior to patient enrollment.

Dr. Burzynski has extensive experience treating cancer with combinations of targeted agents and immunotherapy, and the drug phenylbutyrate (PB), which targets multiple genetic abnormalities simultaneously.

Dr. Burzynski is the author/co-author of over 300 scientific publication/presentations. He has collaborated with investigators at the NCI, the Medical College of Georgia, the Imperial

College of Science and Technology of London, the University of Kurume Medical School in Japan, and the University of Turin Medical School in Italy, among others. He is a member of several prestigious organizations, including the American Medical Association, American Association of Cancer Research (AACR), American Society of Clinical Oncology, the Society for Neuroscience, the Society for Neuro-oncology, the Royal Medical Association (U.K.), and the Academy of Medical Ethics. As of June 2015, he held 245 patents in 35 countries covering his scientific inventions.

Medical maverick, Stanislaw Burzynski, MD, PhD, who has helped cure terminal cancer patients with a non-toxic gene-targeted cancer therapy he developed, is, yet again, under attack. After a decade-long attempt to revoke the cancer pioneer's medical license, which resulted in a Texas Supreme Court victory for Burzynski in 1996, the Texas Medical Board again tried to stop Burzynski from continuing his cancer treatment trials. In 2012 Federal regulators lifted Burzynski's ban and he was allowed to continue his cancer trials.

Antineoplastons and Cancer

Burzynski first discovered antineoplastons, which are peptides and amino acid derivatives that are native to the human body (they are found in blood and urine, but reproduced synthetically for medicinal use), in 1967. He identified that these peptides could control cancer growth, as well as that cancer patients are usually deficient in these peptides, as compared with healthy people.

Antineoplastons are gene-targeted therapeutic agents which activate genes that suppress tumor development and deactivate genes that encourage cancer. Essentially, antineoplastons "reprogram" cancer cells to act like normal cells and die off. Like the many conventional cancer drugs and treatments currently available, antineoplastons cannot promise a cure for all patients; they tend to be more effective against brain cancer and lymphoma, and less effective against lung and breast cancers, and most end-stage cancers.

Unlike chemotherapy and radiation, however, which kill all localized cells – cancerous and healthy – antineoplastons only target cancer cells, and do not harm healthy cells. Hence, they stand to become a mainstream non-toxic alternative in the treatment of some cancers if FDA approved.

FDA Approval of Antineoplastons

Getting antineoplaston therapy approved by the FDA has been an excruciating process so far. While pharmaceutical companies are generally able to get their cancer drugs market-ready within a few months, Dr. Burzynski has fought for decades to get the FDA to sanction his antineoplaston treatment, and against the most ruthless of opposition.

Between 1985 and 1995, the FDA convened five grand jury investigations to indict Burzynski, which, if successful, would have resulted in the closure of his clinic and his going to prison. After four grand juries found the doctor innocent, the FDA finally succeeded in indicting Burzynski on attempt number five. However, after two trials, Burzynski was again found not at fault by the juries. Could Burzynski truly be so savvy that he can fool everyone but the FDA?

Burzynski's patients, whose survival depended on continued antineoplaston treatment, testified on their doctor's behalf throughout the prosecutions. Pressure from Congress and the public eventually forced the FDA to allow Burzynski to continue conducting clinical trials with antineoplastons despite a pending indictment. In 2004, the FDA explicitly acknowledged the potential of antineoplaston treatment as a cancer therapy in 2004 when it granted Orphan Drug status to two types of antineoplastons.

As this point, Burzynski's antineoplaston treatment for recurrent brain stem glioma (which affects children in 80 percent of cases) has completed phase II of the clinical trial process. Now the FDA has thrown another heart wrenching cog into the approval machine by mandating that patients who participate in the phase III trials must also receive radiation treatments together with antineoplaston treatments. Documentary film director Eric Mercola reports that the FDA justified this requirement by stating, "It would be unethical not to give radiation treatment to these patients."

To elucidate the mind-boggling nature of the FDA's radiation mandate, Mercola states:

"Most of the patients to be placed in these trials suffer from inoperable brain cancer. It has been firmly established, based on sound scientific evidence, that radiation treatment administered to the head can not only promote the growth of cancer, but it can result in "brain necrosis," often killing the patient within one or two years after treatment… No hospital in the USA is allowing these Phase 3 antineoplaston "randomized" trials to be conducted, because they know they will never accrue a single patient due to [forced] radiation…What parent would put their child through that? Would you? The FDA does not at all care that the antineoplaston therapy has cured an upward of 30 percent of patients treated of this disease without the inclusion of radiation…[the agency knows] radiation is not necessary to cure any of these kids while using antineoplastons."

The National Cancer Institute at the National Institutes of Health (NIH) even states on various web pages:

"Conventional treatment for children with diffuse intrinsic pontine glioma (DIPG) is radiation therapy to involved areas. Such treatment will result in transient benefit for most patients, but over 90 percent of patients will die within 18 months of diagnosis…. Currently, no chemotherapeutic strategy…when added to radiation therapy has led to long-term survival for children with DIPG."

"Given the dismal prognosis for patients with diffuse intrinsic pontine glioma…Patients should be considered for entry into trials of novel therapeutic approaches because there are no standard agents that have demonstrated a clinically significant activity."

In other words, radiation and chemotherapy have, so far, proved ineffective to treat patients with brain gliomas who could potentially participate in Burzynski's phase III trials. How, then, could it possibly be unethical to not treat patients with radiation, an agent that ultimately leads to death in 90 percent of cases?

In Burzynski's 2003 and 2006 phase II studies, where radiation was not employed, survival 2 years after treatment with antineoplastons (not cancer diagnosis) was 33.3 and 39 percent, respectively; survival 5 years after treatment was, respectively, 17 and 22 percent. Clearly, antineoplaston treatment has shown promise to be more effective against brain stem glioma than radiation, yet the FDA is forcing all Burzynski's phase III trial participants to receive radiation treatments which generally cause more damage than good. Essentially, the FDA is not even giving Burzynski's patients a fighting chance against their cancers, and is not allowing

Burzynski the opportunity to demonstrate just how much more effective antineoplastons may be against cancer than "standard agents."

Connecting the Dots

Without exploring possible ulterior motives the FDA might have for trying to prevent public access to a potential lifesaving and non-toxic cancer therapy, looking at the following bits of information may shine light on the situation at hand:

Cancer treatment is big business. The NIH estimates that the direct medical costs of cancer surpassed $100 billion in 2010.

Chemotherapy, radiation and surgery are the "standard" cancer treatments; chemotherapy and radiation are usually employed when cancer is inoperable.

Pharmaceutical companies and oncologists derive obscene profits from chemotherapy agents and drugs prescribed to counteract their side effects. The system through which oncologists purchase cancer treatments from pharmaceutical companies, then bill insurance companies and Medicare at much higher rates, is said to encourage the overuse of chemotherapy and other expensive drugs, and to override any incentive to find better treatments or a cancer cure.

In 2007, a federal judge in Boston ordered AstraZeneca and Bristol-Myers Squibb to pay almost $14 million in damages for overcharging on cancer drugs (legal analysts have called it a test case for a nationwide class action suit involving Amgen, Abbot Labs and ten other drug companies).

Approval of Burzynski's antineoplaston treatment would represent a change in the pharmaceutical cartel status quo, as a biochemist physician and his small biopharmaceutical company would hold exclusive patent and distribution rights on a paradigm-shifting cancer breakthrough treatment. If a physician and scientist were to own rights to a non-toxic alternative treatment, major pharmaceutical companies would stand to lose serious profits.

In 1982, FDA Bureau of Drugs Director Richard Crout was quoted as saying, **"I never have and never will approve a new drug to an individual, but only to a large pharmaceutical firm with unlimited finances."**

The FDA has been accused before of protecting cancer drug profits. In the May 14, 2007 Wall Street Journal, Mark Thorton, MD, PhD, a former FDA official in the Office of Oncology Products, denounced the FDA's refusal to approve Provenge, a new immunotherapy vaccine for prostate cancer, citing that "the FDA succeeded in killing not one but two safe, promising therapies designed and developed to act by stimulating a patient's immune system against cancer."

Commenting on Thorton's statements, journalist Evelyn Pringle wrote:

"New therapies pose a grave threat to the cancer industry as a whole, and the lost profits would not be limited to the sale of products. The pharmaceutical giants have spent a small fortune to gain control of every segment of the industry, from researchers to government regulators…the profits up for grabs have become so enormous that critics say the goal of industry-controlled research is no longer focused on finding a cure for cancer to save lives. Instead, the focus is on thwarting the development and approval of new therapies in order to protect the profits of the treatments already on the market."

Congress has, in the past, found that FDA advisory committee members with financial ties to pharmaceutical companies (ownership of company stock or patent rights to certain treatments) have had such conflicts of interest waived during approval processes.

Nine FDA scientists wrote this letter to a White House official, urging change at the "fundamentally broken" FDA with information about corruption and distortion in the scientific review process by FDA managers.

While the FDA is handicapping Burzynski by forcing all of his phase III clinical trial patients to undergo radiation treatment, it has given accelerated approval (i.e. mandated completion of phase II only) for a number of drugs manufactured by major pharmaceutical companies that are less effective against brain cancer than antineoplaston treatments.

Hitler's Gift to the World - A Cure for Cancer

Believe it or not Adolf Hitler did one good thing. Hitler's mother died of breast cancer. He himself was paranoid about getting cancer. In the 1930s, when he came to power, he commandeered the top scientists in Germany to find the cure for cancer. In 1931, Dr. Otto Warburg won a Noble Prize in Physiology for his discovery of the cause of cancer. What Dr. Warburg discovered was the fact that when oxygen levels dropped by 35% in a cell it triggered off a process of fermentation just like in the process of making beer and wine. In reality, fermentation was a **survival mechanism, NOT a disease,** that converted glucose to lactic acid to form energy. This process acidified the cells lowing the oxygen levels even more and created the perfect storm for cancer to form. Why do we not hear of Dr. Warburg's research. Follow the money.

If traditional cancer treatments are so successful, why has the FDA, AMA, and the pharmaceutical cartel made a concerted effort to eliminate the competition. There is an outrageous number of physician deaths associated with the suppression of alternative cancer therapies. Why is there no government investigations?

CHAPTER 3

REAL CAUSES OF CANCER

What most people including cancer specialists do not know is that the average newborn today has a minimum of 287 different chemicals in their blood at birth. Of the 287 chemicals that were detected in umbilical cord blood, it is known that 180 cause cancer in humans or animals, 217 are toxic to the brain and nervous system, and 208 cause birth defects or abnormal development in animal tests. The dangers of pre- or post-natal exposure to this complex mixture of carcinogens, developmental toxins and neurotoxins have never been studied. This fact was scientifically documented (published July 14, 2005: www.ewg.org/research/body-burden-pollution-newborns) by the Environmental Working Group (www.ewg.org) who spent $50,000 dollars on each of ten newborn babies. They removed the blood from the placenta at the time of birth and had it analyzed. Their discovery scientifically proved that our environment is so toxic that babies in utero for nine months are being bathed in toxic amniotic fluid. Not long ago scientists thought that the placenta shielded cord blood — and the developing baby — from most chemicals and pollutants in the environment. But now we know that at this critical time when organs, vessels, membranes and systems are knit together from single cells to finished form in a span of weeks, the umbilical cord carries not only the building blocks of life, but also a steady stream of industrial chemicals, pollutants and pesticides that cross the placenta as readily as residues from cigarettes and alcohol. This is the human "body burden" — the pollution in people that permeates everyone in the world, including babies in the womb.

To add insult to injury, these innocent babies are then inoculated with hepatitis B vaccine soon after birth. The baby's blood brain barrier does not mature until eighteen months after birth and is now exposed to the many toxic adjuvants present in the vaccines. Robert F. Kennedy, Jr. has reported that studies done by the vaccine manufactures showed that babies inoculated with the hepatitis B vaccine soon after birth had an 1135% increased chance of becoming autistic. A secret meeting was held in June of 2000 at the Simpsonwood conference center in Norcross, Georgia by NIH, FDA, CDC, WHO, and the four major vaccine manufactures. The purpose of the meeting was to discuss how they were going to keep the lid on the fact that the mercury preservative (Thimerosal) in the hep B vaccine was the cause for autism and how they could hide this information from the public.

Chemical Exposure Sets the Stage for Cancer

The stage has already been set from in utero onward that exposure to numerous initiating factors will eventually cause cancer. It is not a matter if people will get cancer, it is a matter of when they will succumb to cancer. Cancer is **NOT** a disease but an adaptation to the toxins and designed to protect the body.

Ground Breaking Research by Dr. William F. Koch

Dr. William F. Koch, MD, PhD describes three factors in the production of cancer; a **disposing factor,** which is responsible for the anoxia or low oxygen, an **initiating carcinogen**, and a **supportive or propagative carcinogen.**

Disposing Factor

The disposing factor is a fungus found in all specimens of cancer. Dr. Glover identified it in 1923. Dr. Koch found it in 1942. Dr. Irene Diller, a leading bacteriologist at the University of Pennsylvania, identified it in 1948. So it is well identified and, as Dr. Koch claims, its by-product, an amine quite similar to the amines of the antibiotic class used so widely in medicine that causes the gelation of the blood in the area that develops cancer as well as in the general circulation, and this brings about the anoxia required for the further evolution of the pathogenic process.

Initiating Carcinogen

The initiating carcinogen is described by Dr. Koch as quite often a bacterial, nitrogenous product, amines and mercaptans, sulfhydryl compounds that are easily concentrated to form a free radical that integrates into the mitochondrial energy mechanism. This chain of events diminishes the little power house's (mitochondria) ability to produce ATP (adenosine triphosphate) to run the functions of the cell.

Supportive or Propagative Carcinogen

When oxygen is lacking, the free radical formed by the dehydrogenation (a chemical reaction that involves the removal of hydrogen from an organic molecule) cannot combine oxygen and form a peroxide free radical to continue the combustion process (which destroys the cancer initiating factors). This free radical can do only one thing, and that is add to the closest double bond at hand, and this double bond is the very one that binds with and activates the Carbonyl group which removed its hydrogen atom to form the free radical. Thereby the foreign substance, or fuel product, is integrated with the host's mitochondria (power house of the cell) and paralyzes its energy production, and normal function is blocked. However, the function can be forced beyond physiological control by receiving vicarious energy (from fermentation - occurs in a low oxygen environment) as the result of the following events, and thereby the various allergies and cancer can come about. Viruses are initiating carcinogens that require the cooperation of the polymerizing bacterial products (amines) to complete the act of cancer production.

The concept that Dr. Koch offers, focuses on a **Least Common Denominator** in, pathogenesis, which is based on the properties of the double bond methylene groups and the free radical. He uses these same properties to accomplish an orderly reversal of the pathogenesis.

The Koch's Concept exhibits some of the features of homeopathy, and is constructive and corrective. Thus, in the performance of this therapy, germs and viruses are not killed but are changed to their normal non-pathogenic status. Cancer cells are relieved of their injurious factor and are given the chance to reconstruct to normalcy; the paralyzed nerve cells are cleared of the virus that has blocked their physiology so the cell is free to perform its normal functions again. Dr. Koch has used this circumstance to prove that the virus that had integrated with the nerve cell is actually removed, because as long as the virus occupies the vital positions within the cell, the cell function is paralyzed, and when function returns the virus must be absent.

It is well known too that once a virus penetrates a cell, that cell is doomed, since **no known orthodox system of treatment** can separate the virus from the vital part of the host cell by any amount of anti-toxic serum, vaccines, or other measure of that kind. This is because the atomic bonding between the host cell and the virus are so firm that once the integration is made it cannot be broken by any orthodox means. This firm integration between the virus and the cell takes place within one and a half minutes after the virus has penetrated.

Dr. Koch's research was performed back in the mid-1920s. His discoveries are as true today as they were back then. The big difference was the fact that during that period our environment was not as toxic, our food was more vital, and we didn't have dental titanium implants or root canal treatments; we didn't have chemtrail pollution; we didn't have much in the way of electromagnetic frequency issues and vaccinations were not mandatory and there were very few if any. We also didn't have the ubiquitous cancer causing glyphosate (Monsanto's Roundup) laced in our food, air and rain water.

Today there are so many carcinogenic variables assaulting our body and in my professional opinion the reason why we have so much cancer among our population. An additional problem exists in the fact that most healthcare practitioners do not have the skills or knowledge to diagnose the presence of heavy metals, residual dental infections, stealth viruses, bacteria, fungi, mold, glyphosate, and thousands of pesticides, insecticides, and herbicides that confront patients.

A perfect example of what Dr. Koch was referring to was observed in a 17 year-old male patient who was diagnosed by conventional medicine with osteosarcoma (cancer of the skeletal muscle and bone). The oncologic surgeon basically mutilated this boy's leg by cutting out the cancer (part of the leg muscle and femur bone). This patient was referred to my practice. The boy presented with constant pain in the cancer site. Traditional medicine with all its sophisticated blood testing, CT scans and MRIs could not decipher the cause of the patient's chronic pain. Using Quantum Testing Techniques on the pathology slides of the patient's cancer, the cancerous tissue was contaminated with aluminum, cadmium, mercury, glyphosate, and cytomegalovirus. A customized nutritional program was formulated to remove the initiators. When the patient returned six weeks later, his chronic pain was totally resolved. Also of significance was the fact that when the glyphosate was removed with a homeopathic remedy, all his allergies disappeared. Over the course of two years, the remaining "splinters" were removed and the patient's cancer was put into remission.

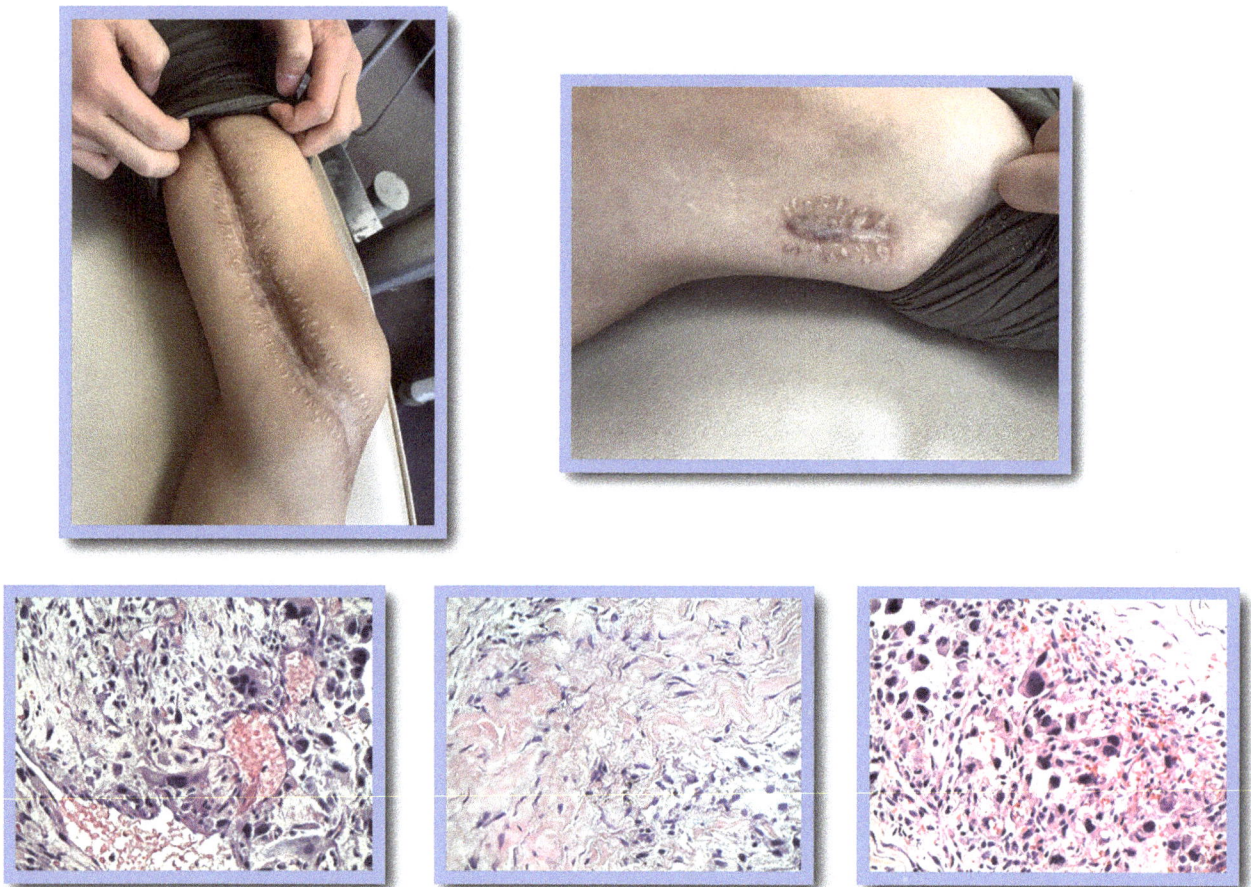

Figure 1. Surgical mutilation. Cutting out the cancer is not the solution. Removing the "splinters" is the solution. Changing the terrain, removing the initiators, raising the oxygen level of the cells, and rebalancing the energies creates an environment in which cancer cannot grow.

Quantum Testing Technique developed by this author defined the initiators in the cancerous tissue as presented in the pathology slides. Aluminum, cadmium, mercury, cytomegalovirus, and glyphosate were the "splinters" or initiators that caused the cancer. Conventional oncologic concepts have no clue as to this innovative technology nor do they understand the true nature of cancer. All they know is "kill" the cancer and treat the symptoms. This paradigm is obsolete.

Another example of Dr. Koch's three components of cancer (Deposing Factor, Initiating Carcinogen, and the Supportive or propagating Carcinogen) is exhibited in a 72 year-old stage IV throat cancer patient. Conventional medicine wanted to surgically remove the cancer in his throat, which would have mutilated the patient and required him to have a feeding tube for the rest o this life. This represents the gold standard in oncology today. Faced with the prospect of being permanently disfigured and a feeding tube, the patient opted for an alternative approach that was less invasive.

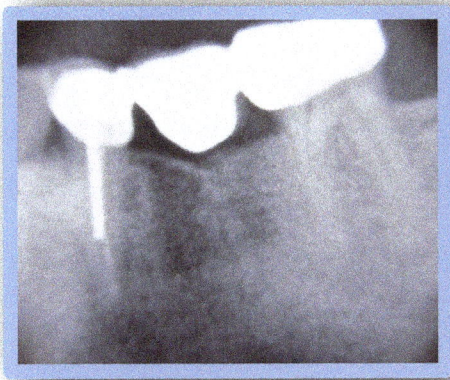

Figure 2.

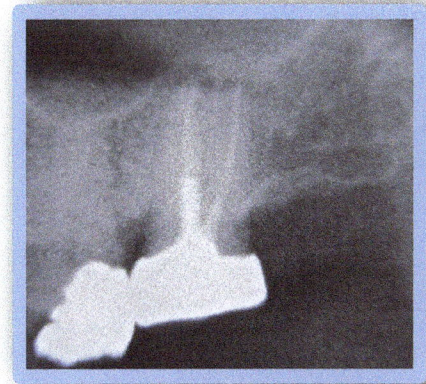

Comprehensive evaluation revealed two root canal treated teeth and one with a necrotic (dead) pulp. Using the Quantum Testing Technique, *Streptococcus viridans* and *Tuberculinum* were diagnosed in the root canal treated teeth. These were the same pathogens that were present in the area of the throat cancer. Interestingly, when the patient told his endocrinologist that he was going to seek alternative therapies, the physician told him alternative therapy is a farce and a waste of time and money. Three weeks after the two root canal teeth and one necrotic tooth were removed and the surgical sites ozonated and irrigated with colloidal silver and homeopathic remedies and complemented with Rife frequency treatment, Insulin Potentiation therapy, raw food diet and supplements, the cancer disappeared. When the patient confronted his doctor and asked him if he could speak with his other cancer patients, the endocrinologist refused to speak with him. You instinctively know that the conventional medical system is broken when the "doctor" refuses to entertain alternative therapies that work.

Figure 2. Root canal treated teeth represent dead organs which in a high percentage of cases become infected and spew out toxic chemicals like mercaptans, thioethers, and hydrogen sulfide. When the teeth were removed, the source of the cancer initiators was removed and the cancer was able to revert back to normal tissue. This basic concept is not part of oncologist's knowledge base because it is not taught in the medical schools.

The infections and toxins drain through the lymphatic system to contaminate the throat. Most cancer specialists do not consider the teeth as potential sources for causing cancer.

Another Case in Point

Lung cancer is one of the more difficult cancers to cure especially when it metastasizes. This was the case of a 56 year-old female who was diagnosed with carcinoma of the right lung. The gold standard of treatment was cut the tip of the right lung off where the cancer was located. Unfortunately for this patient, the cancer returned in six months in the upper part of her left lung. The patient stated that "she would rather die than go through the surgery again." The patient was referred to my office for evaluation and treatment. The patients' dental x-rays revealed a root canal tooth in the lower left side of her jaw. Interestingly, the tooth was infected with CMV (cytomegalovirus). This same virus that was also present in the hospital's pathology slides of the cancer.

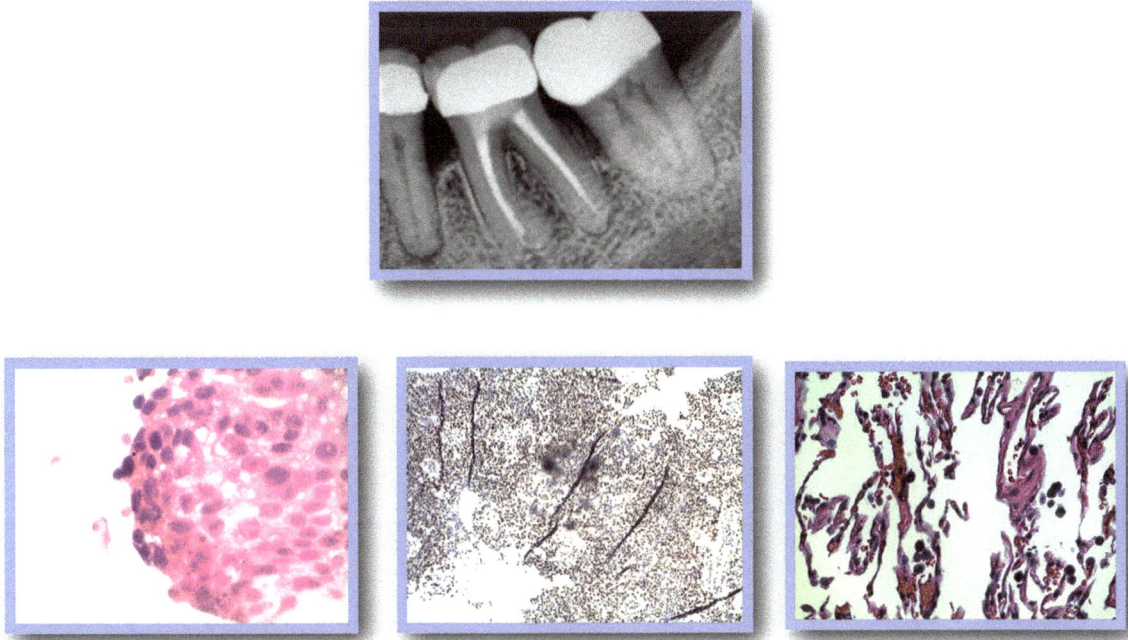

Figure 3. The lower left first molar root canal tooth was infected with CMV, which was the same pathogen in the cancer tissue in the lung.

Quantum Testing Diagnosed: CMV, Hg, and a pesticide in the cancerous tissue. This is one of the major missing links in treatment of cancer today. Very few practitioners are defining the causative factors.

In addition to the CMV, there was mercury and a pesticide in the cancer tissue. Six months after the patient was placed on food based supplements to remove the three "splinters" the cancer disappeared. Once again the body in its infinite wisdom will to go back to "factory default" when the cancer initiators are removed. These three cases validate Dr. Koch's concepts on the cause of cancer and the ability for cancer cells to transition back to normal.

Dental Cancer Connection

Be cautious of old barbers and young dentists. Comprehensive dentistry has its pitfalls. Unfortunately, most dentists are not aware that residual infections in the bone can occur even after failed root canal or abscessed teeth are removed. Replacement implants are put into infected bone and they do not even know it. The problem is that ALL structures in the mouth are drained by the lymphatic system into the throat, neck area, thyroid, thymus, breasts and elsewhere. This was the case with a patient who spent 80 thousand plus dollars to have implants and bridgework placed to restore his missing teeth.

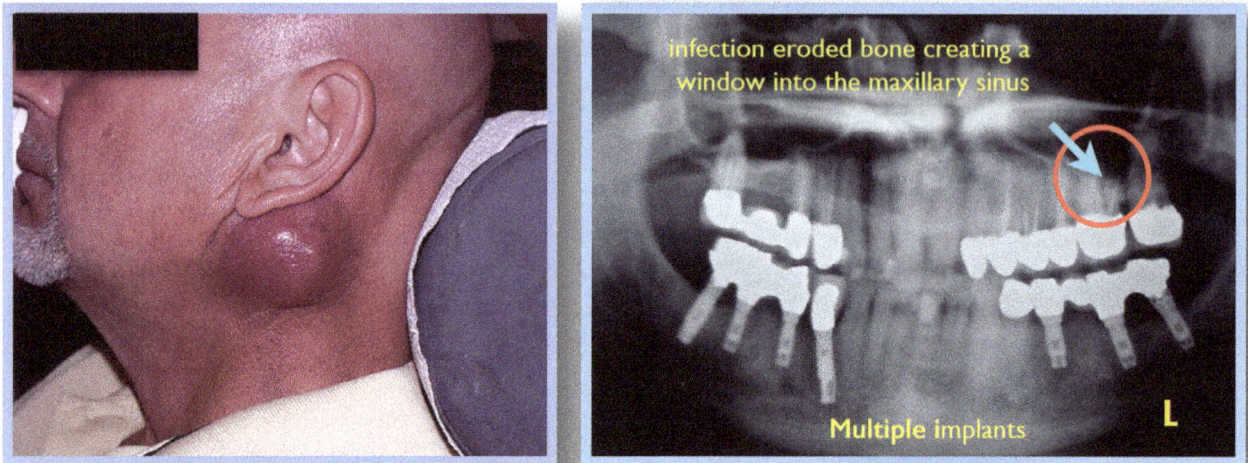

Figure 4. Multiple root canals, which represent dead organs create chronic inflammation and provide a source for multiple pathogens and chemical toxins like mercaptans, thioethers, and hydrogen sulfide. These toxins drain into the neck area and beyond. Quantum Testing determined that the same pathogens that were in the patient's infected root canal treated teeth were in the neck tumor.

In addition, the multiple titanium implants plus gold and porcelain crowns create low level galvanic (electric) currents in the mouth impacting normal cell function. Remember cancer is an adaptation not a disease. The corrupted DNA and organelles within cells over grow to assimilate the continuous flow of toxins.

Common Potential Carcinogenic Initiators

This list provides the main categories that have to be tested. Each of the categories has literally thousands of items that can be evaluated. This is where conventional medicine falls way short of the mark. Blood tests will not pick up these carcinogens especially if they are trapped within cells, organs, or tissues. This is also the reason why today's conventional medicine is obsolete. The findings that blood test reveal are reactions to the initiators and they do not reveal the causative factors.

- **Heavy metals:** the most common ones found in cancer patients are: mercury, aluminum, arsenic, cadmium, lead, and nickel.
- **Infections:** common ones found are cytomegalovirus, Epstein Barr virus, *Streptococcus viridans,* fungi, molds, herpes zoster (shingles), herpes simplex I & II, and candida.
- **Chemicals:** most common ones are dioxins, benzene, pesticides, insecticides, and herbicides, especially glyphosate.
- **Parasites:** most common ones found are giardia, cryptosporidium, flukes, pin worms, tapeworms, and amoebas; schistosoma haematobium (squamous cell carcinoma of the bladder).
- **Vaccines and their adjuvants:** most common ones are tetanus, MMR, gardasil, chicken pox, meningococcal, thimerosal (neurotoxin), aluminum (neurotoxin), flu, pertussis, and diphtheria; adjuvants such as formaldehyde, polysorbate 80, thimerosal (ethyl mercury), retro virus contamination (SV40 - simian virus 40 from monkey kidneys), and cell lines, which are derived from aborted human babies which can mutate into cancer causing agents. Nagalase has also been found in vaccines, which is known to suppress the body's immune system.
- **Cancer Causing Foods:** refined sugar, soda (high fructose corn syrup plus chemical additives), processed meats, red meats (chemicalized: hormones, antibiotics, steroids), microwave popcorn, herbicide laden fruits and vegetables, potato chips (high temperature cooking creates the compound acrylamide), farmed raised fish (fed chemicals to give the reddish-pink hue, antibiotics and pesticides, which are also well-known carcinogens), canned foods are contaminated with bisphenol-A or BPA form the plastic lining in the cans, hydrogenated oils (chemically processed for longer shelf-life), refined white flour (stripped of all its nutrients), alcohol, genetically modified foods, artificial sweeteners (Equal*, Splenda, Sweet'N Low), diet products with artificial chemicals, smoked meats (smoking process retains large amounts of hazardous tar, known to be a carcinogen), and foods high in estrogen (soy and flax seeds, which have three times the amount of phytoestrogen than soy).

Note: *Equal (Aspartame) breaks down in the body to formaldehyde (cancer causing), formic acid, and methanol, which can make you go blind.

Carcinogens and Mechanisms Causing Cancer

There are many mechanisms that can trigger off cancer. Some of the processes are more notable and others are obscure. The key to keep in mind is the fact that by removing the "splinters" or initiators the cancer cells can return to normal function. Remember that cancer is **NOT** a disease but a **survival mechanism**; when the body's environment becomes polluted and cellular oxygen is reduced by 35%, the cell organelles get dysfunctional especially the mitochondria and cells start dividing to compensate for these abnormal conditions. As a result of 10 years of laboratory experiments at the University of Michigan and at the Detroit College of Medicine and of 7 years of clinical observation, Dr. Koch, MD, PhD concludes that cancer is a systemic disease of parasitic origin, that the cancer tumor is an inadequate effort on the part of nature against the toxins of the invading organism and that cancer can be cured.

- Carcinogenic compounds induce chromosomal abnormalities and DNA strand breakage occurs.
- Mercury gives off between 13 and 21 different frequencies; once inside the cell these frequencies disrupt the normal physiology of the organelles. Mercury leaks out of amalgam fillings in teeth 24/7; its present in many fish and as a preservative in vaccines (Thimerosal). It's a neurotoxin along with aluminum, which is another vaccine preservative.
- In the 1970s, a German researcher by the name of Dr. Fritz Albert Popp discovered that carcinogens, like mercury, dioxin or any other one, prevents the body from absorbing the wavelength of 380 nm, which prevents repair of the DNA. This effect holds true for all carcinogens.
- Nagalase is a protein excreted by cancer cells and viruses in the body. It prevents the naturally occurring immune booster, Globulin component Macrophage Activating Factor (GcMAF), from being produced by the liver. Nagalase also suppresses vitamin

D_3, which suppresses the immune system. Nagalase has been found as a contaminant in many vaccines.

- Hypothyroidism creates excess mucopolysaccharides within the interstitial tissues and in turn causes inflammation and edema. In addition, a low functioning thyroid also reduces the metabolism of cells, which causes a build up of metabolic wastes. An underactive thyroid also weakens the immune system.

- Adulterated oils (safflower, sunflower, corn, soy, walnut, canola, cottonseed) which are present in our snack foods, bottled oils at the supper market, and most prepared foods, corrupt the cell membrane by turning it into plastic. It is the adulterated omega 6 and omega 3 oils that are pro inflammatory and prevent the uptake of oxygen and nutrients from entering the cell and waste products from exiting. This phenomenon is one of the basic factors aging our body and causing widespread degenerative diseases.

- Consumption of high doses of fish oil increases the risk of colon cancer (Fenton, J, et al., "Link Between Fish Oil and Increased Risk of Colon Cancer in Mice," Medical news Today (Colorectal Cancer), article URL: www.medicalnewstoday. com/articles/203683.php#post, October 7, 2010

- Medical News Today reported on a study (back in the 1960s) that showed that over half of mice fed a sucrose-rich diet developed breast cancer. The study revealed that the mice fed a diet high in sucrose had a lower level of beta-glucuronidase, which is a protective enzyme with potent hepatoprotective effect against carbon tetrachloride (CCl4) induced liver injury. Consumption of sugar elevates insulin levels, which causes systemic inflammation. Inflammation causes scarring, which impedes blood flow and results in a buildup of toxins creating a pathological terrain.

D H Kim 1, S B Shim, N J Kim, I S Jang: Beta-glucuronidase-inhibitory activity and hepatoprotective effect of Ganoderma lucidum. Bio Pharm Bull. 1999 Feb; 22(2):162-4. doi: 10.1248/bpb.22.162.

Cell Membrane Potential and Cancer Progression

Membrane potential (Vm), the voltage across the cell plasma membrane, arises because of the presence of different ion channels/transporters with specific ion selectivity and permeability. Cell membrane potential is a key biophysical signal modulating important cellular activity, such as proliferation and differentiation. The cell membrane potential is directly influenced by the various ion channels/transporters that fine tune and regulate the cell membrane potential. The intracellular Na+ level is markedly higher in tumors compared to non-cancerous tissues, whereas the K+ level remains more stable (Smith et al., 1978; Cameron et al., 1980; Sparks et al., 1983). An increased intracellular Na+ concentration could be a determinant of depolarized rapidly cycling cancer cells. It is well-established that cancer cells possess distinct bioelectrical properties. ***When the cell membrane potential drops from a -70 mV (healthy cell - oral pH 7.43) to a + 55 mV (pathological voltage - oral pH 5.24) it is a prerequisite to trigger off cell proliferation. At the pathological voltage of +55 mV, the DNA gets damaged and cancer forms.*** Interestingly, there is no cell division above -20 mV and viruses, bacteria, fungi, and cancer cells die between a cell pH of 7.8 to 8.8. Human blood has a pH range of 7.35 to 7.5 and corresponds to a cell membrane potential between -20 to -30 millivolts respectively. The millivolts to pH relationship was first discovered by Dr. Jerry Tennant.

These same ion channels/transporters control cell volume and migration. This depolarization or drop in cell membrane potential has a functional role in cancer cell metastasis. Because of a lack of energy (mitochondrial dysfunction) cancer cells cannot increase membrane potential so they remain in the proliferation stage all the time. The lower the cell membrane potential the higher the rate of cancer cell growth.

Front Physiol
2013 Jul 17;4:185. doi: 10.3389/fphys.2013.00185. eCollection 2013.
Membrane potential and cancer progression
PMID: 23882223 PMCID: PMC3713347 DOI: 10.3389/fphys.2013.00185

To achieve healing, a state of hyperpolarization is required for stem cell differentiation in order to repair cells. As an example, osteogenesis, formation of new bone, is hindered in human mesenchymal stem cells (primitive cells that can form muscles, bone, tendons, lung, etc.) under depolarizing conditions. Regarding cancer, membrane depolarization might be important for the emergence and maintenance of cancer stem cells (CSCs), giving rise to sustained tumor growth. From a treatment perspective, cutting out the cancer, irradiating it, or "killing" the cancer with chemotherapy does **NOT** correct the cell membrane potential or any other cancer initiating factors. The stage is set for a recurrence which often occurs.

Membrane potentials within cells are determined primarily by three factors: 1) the concentration of potassium ions on the inside and sodium ions outside of the cell; 2) the permeability (corrupt cell membranes from adulterated omega 6 oils impede permeability) of the cell membrane to those ions (i.e., ion conductance) through specific ion channels; and 3) by the activity of electrogenic pumps (e.g., Na + /K + -Adenosine Triphosphatase and Ca ++ transport pumps) that maintain the ion concentrations across the membrane.

The Redox signaling (a process in which one substance or molecule is reduced and the other is oxidized) molecules whose primary source are mitochondria have a direct effect on gene expression, apoptosis (cell death), cell growth, cell adhesion, chemotaxis (characteristic movement of an organism or cell along a chemical concentration gradient either toward or away from the chemical stimulus) angiogenesis (growth of new blood vessels), immune reactions, and inflammation. Exposure to carcinogens, benzene, fluoride, mercury, glyphosate, etc. directly affects the various organelles within the cell especially mitochondria. Mitochondria are responsible for:

- Energy production
- Cellular respiration
- Cellular energy production
- Calcium homeostasis
- Cell growth
- Cell death
- Oxidative radical regulation
- Nerve conduction
- Synthesis of bio-molecules
- Role in disease
- Metabolism

Mitochondria play a major role as a cell dispatcher; they orchestrate the functions within the cell. When patients complain of fatigue, it is caused by toxicity of these organelles.

Comprehensive cancer treatment must include detoxing the body especially the mitochondria. If the foundational issues, cell membrane potential, corrupt cell membranes, cell toxicity, acid pH, mineral deficiencies, and others are not addressed, it is virtually impossible to reverse the cancer.

Mammograms Cause Cancer

Breast cancer is the leading cause of death among American women between the ages of 44 and 55. Dr. Gofinan, in his book, *Preventing Breast Cancer*, cites this startling statistic along with an in-depth look at mammographic screening, an early-detection practice that agencies like the American Cancer Society recommend to women of all age groups. According to most health experts, catching a tumor in its early stages increases a woman's chances of survival by at least 17 percent.

The most common method for early detection is mammography. A mammogram is an X-ray picture of your breast that can reveal tumor growths otherwise undetectable in a physical exam. Like all x-rays, mammograms use doses of ionizing radiation to create this image. Radiologists then analyze the image for any abnormal growths. Despite continuous improvements and innovations, mammography has garnered a sizable opposition in the medical community because of an error rate that is still high and the amount of harmful radiation used in the procedure.

Effectiveness of Mammography

Is mammography an effective tool for detecting tumors? Some critics say no. In a Swedish study of 60,000 women, 70 percent of the mammographically detected tumors weren't tumors at all. These "false positives" aren't just financial and emotional strains, they may also lead to many unnecessary and invasive biopsies. In fact, 70 to 80 percent of all positive mammograms do not, upon biopsy, show any presence of cancer.

At the same time, mammograms also have a high rate of missed tumors, or "false negatives." Dr. Samuel S. Epstein, in his book, *The Politics Of Cancer*, claims that in women ages 40 to

49, one in four instances of cancer is missed at each mammography. The National Cancer Institute (NCI) puts the false negative rate even higher at 40 percent among women ages 40-49. National Institutes of Health spokespeople also admit that mammograms miss 10 percent of malignant tumors in women over 50. Researchers have found that breast tissue is denser among younger women, making it difficult to detect tumors. For this reason, false negatives are twice as likely to occur in premenopausal mammograms.

Radiation Risks

Many critics of mammography cite the hazardous health effects of radiation. In 1976, the controversy over radiation and mammography reached a saturation point. At that time mammographic technology delivered five to 10 rads (radiation-absorbed doses) per screening, as compared to 1 rad in current screening methods. In women between the ages of 35 and 50, each rad of exposure increased the risk of breast cancer by one percent, according to Dr. Frank Rauscher, then-director of the National Cancer Institute.

According to the well respected neurosurgeon, Russell L. Blaylock, MD, one estimate is that annual radiological breast exams increase the risk of breast cancer by two percent a year. So over 10 years the risk will have increased 20 percent. In the 1960s and 70s, women, even those who received 10 screenings, were never told the risk they faced from exposure. In the midst of the 1976 radiation debate, Kodak, a major manufacturer of mammography film, took out full-page ads in scientific journals entitled About breast cancer and X-rays: A hopeful message from industry on a sober topic.

Despite better technology and decreased doses of radiation, scientists still claim mammography is a substantial risk. Dr. John W. Gofman, an authority on the health effects of ionizing radiation, estimates that 75 percent of breast cancer could be prevented by avoiding or minimizing exposure to the ionizing radiation. This includes mammography, x-rays and other medical and dental sources.

Since mammographic screening was introduced, the incidence of a form of breast cancer called ductal carcinoma in situ (DCIS) has increased by 328 percent. Two hundred percent of this increase is allegedly due to mammography. In addition to harmful radiation, mammography may also help spread existing cancer cells due to the considerable pressure placed on the woman's breast during the procedure. According to some health practitioners, this compression could cause existing cancer cells to metastasize from the breast tissue.

Cancer research has also found a gene, called oncogene AC, that is extremely sensitive to even small doses of radiation. A significant percentage of women in the United States have this gene, which could increase their risk of mammography-induced cancer. They estimate that 10,000 A-T (genetic disorder ataxia-telangiectasia) carriers will die of breast cancer this year due to mammography.

The risk of radiation is apparently higher among younger women. The NCI released evidence that, among women under 35, mammography could cause 75 cases of breast cancer for every 15 it identifies. Another Canadian study found a 52 percent increase in breast cancer mortality in young women given annual mammograms. Dr. Samuel Epstein also claims that pregnant women exposed to radiation could endanger their fetus. He advises against mammography during pregnancy because "the future risks of leukemia to your unborn child, not to mention birth defects, are just not worth it." Similarly, studies reveal that children exposed to radiation are more likely to develop breast cancer as adults.

The experts Speak on Mammograms and Breast Cancer:

Regular mammography of younger women increases their cancer risks. Analysis of controlled trials over the last decade has shown consistent increases in breast cancer mortality within a few years of commencing screening. This confirms evidence of the high sensitivity of the premenopausal breast, and on cumulative carcinogenic effects of radiation. *The Politics Of Cancer* by Samuel S Epstein MD, page 539

In his book, *Preventing Breast Cancer*, Dr. Gofinan says that breast cancer is the leading cause of death among American women between the ages of forty-four and fifty-five. Because breast tissue is highly radiation-sensitive, mammograms can cause cancer. The danger can be heightened by a woman's genetic makeup, preexisting benign breast disease, artificial menopause, obesity, and hormonal imbalance. Death By Medicine by Gary Null PhD, page 23

"The risk of radiation-induced breast cancer has long been a concern to mammographers and has driven the efforts to minimize radiation dose per examination," the panel explained. "Radiation can cause breast cancer in women, and the risk is proportional to dose. The younger the woman at the time of exposure, the greater her lifetime risk for breast cancer. *Under The Influence Modern Medicine* by Terry A Rondberg DC, page 122

Furthermore, there is clear evidence that the breast, particularly in premenopausal women, is highly sensitive to radiation, with estimates of increased risk of breast cancer of up to 1% for every rad (radiation absorbed dose) unit of X-ray exposure. This projects up to a 20% increased cancer risk for a woman who, in the 1970s, received 10 annual mammograms of an average two rads each. In spite of this, up to 40% of women over 40 have had mammograms since the mid-1960s, some annually and some with exposures of 5 to 10 rads in a single screening from older, high-dose equipment. *The Politics Of Cancer by Samuel* S Epstein MD, page 537

No less questionable—or controversial—has been the use of X rays to detect breast cancer: mammography. The American Cancer Society initially promoted the procedure as a safe and simple way to detect breast tumors early and thus allow women to undergo mastectomies before their cancers had metastasized. The *Cancer Industry* by Ralph W Moss, page 23

The American Cancer Society, together with the American College of Radiologists, has insisted on pursuing large scale mammography screening programs for breast cancer, including its use in younger women, even though the NCI and other experts now agree that these are likely to cause more cancers than could possibly be detected. *The Politics Of Cancer* by Samuel S Epstein MD, page 291

A number of "cancer societies" argued, saying the tests — which cost between $50-200 each are a necessity for all women over 40, despite the fact that radiation from yearly mammograms during ages 40-49 has been estimated to cause one additional breast cancer death per 10,000 women. *Under The Influence Modern Medicine* by Terry A Rondberg DC, page 21

Mammograms Add to Cancer Risk—mammography exposes the breast to damaging ionizing radiation. John W. Gofman, M.D., Ph.D., an authority on the health effects of ionizing radiation, spent 30 years studying the effects of low-dose radiation on humans. He estimates that 75% of breast cancer could be prevented by avoiding or minimizing exposure to the ionizing radiation from mammography, X rays, and other medical sources. Other research has shown that, during a mammogram, considerable pressure must be placed on the woman's breast, as the breast is squeezed between two flat plastic surfaces. According to some health practitioners, this compression could cause existing cancer cells to metastasize from the breast tissue. *Alternative Medicine* by Burton Goldberg, page 588

In fact the benefits of annual screening to women age 40 to 50, who are now being aggressively recruited, are at best controversial. In this age group, one in four cancers is missed at each mammography. Over a decade of pre-menopausal screening, as many as three in 10 women will be mistakenly diagnosed with breast cancer. Moreover, international studies have shown that routine premenopausal mammography is associated with increased breast cancer death rates at older ages. Factors involved include: the high sensitivity of the premenopausal breast to the cumulative carcinogenic effects of mammographic X-radiation; the still higher sensitivity to radiation of women who carry the A-T gene; and the danger that forceful and often painful compression of the breast during mammography may rupture small blood vessels and encourage distant spread of undetected cancers. *The Politics Of Cancer* by Samuel S Epstein MD, page 540

Since a mammogram is basically an x-ray (radiation) of the breast, I do not recommend mammograms to my patients for two reasons: 1) Few radiologists are able to read mammogams correctly, therefore limiting their effectiveness. Even the man who developed this technique stated on national television that only about six radiologists in the United States could read them correctly. 2) In addition, each time the breasts are exposed to an x-ray, the risk of breast cancer increases by 2 percent. *The Hope of Living Cancer Free* by Francisco Contreras MD, page 104

The use of women as guinea pigs is familiar. There is revealing consistency between the tamoxifen trial and the 1970s trial by the NCI and American Cancer Society involving high-dose mammography of some 300,000 women. Not only is there little evidence of effectiveness of mammography in premenopausal women, despite NCI's assurances no warnings were given of the known high risks of breast cancer from the excessive X-ray doses then used. There has been no investigation of the incidence of breast cancer in these high-risk women.

Of related concern is the NCI's continuing insistence on premenopausal mammography, in spite of contrary warnings by the American College of Physicians and the Canadian Breast Cancer Task Force and in spite of persisting questions about hazards even at current low-dose exposures. These problems are compounded by the NCI's failure to explore safe alternatives, especially transillumination with infrared light scanning. *The Politics Of Cancer* by Samuel S Epstein MD, page 544

"Radiation-related breast cancers occur at least 10 years after exposure," continued the panel. "Radiation from yearly mammograms during ages 40-49 has been estimated to cause one additional breast cancer death per 10,000 women." *Under The Influence Modern Medicine* by Terry A Rondberg DC, page 122

Equivocal mammogram results lead to unnecessary surgery, and the accuracy rate of mammograms is poor. According to the National Cancer Institute (NCI), in women ages 40-49, there is a high rate of "missed tumors," resulting in 40% false-negative mammogram results. *Alternative Medicine* by Burton Goldberg, page 973

It is strongly recommended that you refuse routine mammograms to detect early breast cancer, especially if you are premenopausal. The X-rays may actually increase your chances of getting cancer. If you are older, and there are strong reasons to suspect that you may have breast cancer, the risks may be worthwhile. Very few circumstances, if any, should persuade you to have X-rays taken if you are pregnant. The future risks of leukemia to your unborn child, not to mention birth defects, are just not worth it. *The Politics Of Cancer* by Samuel S Epstein MD, page 305

Because there is no reduction in mortality from breast cancer as a direct result of early mammograms, it is recommended that women under 50 avoid screening mammograms, although the American Cancer Society is still recommending a mammogram every two years for women ages 40-49. The NCI recommends that, after age 35, women perform monthly breast self-exams. For women over 50, many doctors still advocate mammograms. However, breast self-exams and safer, more accurate technologies such as thermography should be strongly considered as options to mammography. *Alternative Medicine* by Burton Goldberg, page 973

The largest and most credible study ever done to evaluate the impact of routine mammography on survival has concluded that routine mammograms do significantly reduce deaths from breast cancer. Scientists in the United States, Sweden, Britain, and Taiwan compared the number of deaths from breast cancer diagnosed in the 20 years before mammogram screening became available with the number in the 20 years after its introduction. The research was based on the histories and treatment of 210,000 Swedish women ages 20 to 69. The researchers found that death from breast cancer dropped 44 percent in women who had routine mammography. Among those who refused mammograms during this time period there was only a 16 percent reduction in death from this disease (presumably the decrease was due to better treatment of the malignancy). Dr Isadore Rosenfeld's *Breakthrough Health* By Isadore Rosenfeld MD, page 47

In 1993—seventeen years after the first pilot study—the biochemist Mary Wolff and her colleagues conducted the first carefully designed, major study on this issue. They analyzed DDE (pesticide - Dichlorodiphenyldichloroethylene) and PCB (polychlorinated biphenyls) levels in the stored blood specimens of 14,290 New York City women who had attended a mammography screening clinic. Within six months, fifty-eight of these women were diagnosed with breast cancer. Wolff matched each of these fifty-eight women to control subjects—women without cancer but of the same age, same menstrual status, and so on—who had also visited the clinic. The blood samples of the women with breast cancer were then compared to their cancer-free counterparts. *Living Downstream* by Sandra Steingraber PhD, page 12

One reason may be that mammograms actually increase mortality. In fact numerous studies to date have shown that among the under-50s, more women die from breast cancer among screened groups than among those not given mammograms. The results of the Canadian National Breast Cancer Screening Trial published in 1993, after a screen of 50,000 women between 40-49, showed that more tumors were detected in the screened group, but not only were no lives saved but 36 percent more women died from breast cancer. *The Cancer Handbook* by Lynne McTaggart, page 57

One Canadian study found a 52 percent increase in breast cancer mortality in young women given annual mammograms, a procedure whose stated purpose is to prevent cancer. Despite evidence of the link between cancer and radiation exposure to women from mammography, the American Cancer Society still promotes the practice without reservation. Five radiologists have served as ACS presidents.53 *When Healing Becomes A Crime* by Kenny Ausubel, page 233

A study reported that mammography combined with physical exams found 3,500 cancers, 42 percent of which could not be detected by physical exam. However, 31 percent of the tumors were non-infiltrating cancer. Since the course of breast cancer is long, the time difference in cancer detected through mammography may not be a benefit in terms of survival. *Woman's Encyclopedia Of Natural Healing* by Dr Gary Null, page 86

For breast cancer, thermography offers a very early warning system, often able to pinpoint a cancer process five years before it would be detectable by mammography. Most breast tumors have been growing slowly for up to 20 years before they are found by typical diagnostic techniques. Thermography can detect cancers when they are at a minute physical stage of development, when it is still relatively easy to halt and reverse the progression of the cancer. No rays of any kind enter the patient's body; there is no pain or compressing of the breasts as in a mammogram. While mammography tends to lose effectiveness with dense breast tissue, thermography is not dependent upon tissue densities. *Alternative Medicine* by Burton Goldberg, page 587

There are a myriad of pathways to form cancer. The information put forth in this book is by no mean the complete story but was designed to wake people up to seek other avenues in their quest to restore their health. The message is clear. Medicine's diagnostic technology itself can cause cancer and is very limited and unfortunately reveals only the reactions to the initiators and not the cause. A perfect example of this is exemplified in a case I treated in 2010. A 62 year-old male patient presented with a medical history of a swollen liver for twenty-seven years. His blood test revealed an elevated alkaline phosphatase level, which is indicative of liver dysfunction. For twenty-seven years medicine's gold standard of testing could not define the underlying cause for Fred's swollen liver. Medicine's answer to his problem was a liver transplant. The patient's response was "thanks but no thanks."

Fred's wife found my website and brought him in for evaluation and treatment. Quantum Testing revealed that Fred's liver was contaminated with two initiators: benzene and hepatitis

B. The patient was placed on a custom nutritional program of food based supplements. In seven months, his swollen liver totally resolved and his alkaline phosphatase level went back to normal. Ironically, Fred has had blood tests every six months for the past ten years. Every blood test revealed a normal liver but his insurance company keeps telling him that he cannot be insured because he has a liver problem. Unfortunately, physicians and the majority of our healthcare industry have been dumbed down so they cannot even recognize the truth.

The next phase after one becomes aware of the potential initiators is how to define them. This is where energy medicine transitions into the new realm of Quantum Medicine. As patients become aware of this latest technology they will seek out practitioners who have the knowledge and skills to solve their health problems.

"The more I meet oncologists, the more I love my cats."
Dr. Gerald H. Smith
Zoey (top) and Nikki

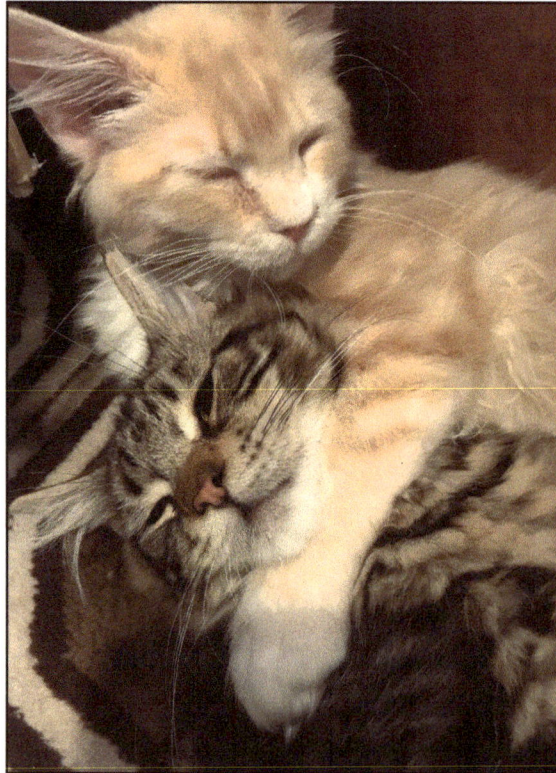

CHAPTER 4

HISTORICAL PERSPECTIVE

The evolution of the Quantum Testing Technique follows an interesting historical path. The following description is a kaleidoscope of events involving pioneer researchers who definitely thought outside of the box. Fortunately for this author many of the geniuses that formulated the many aspects of the Quantum Testing Technique, provided tutelage, which enabled me to hone my testing and diagnostic skills.

Sacro Occipital Technique (SOT)

The journey starts with Major Bertrand DeJarnette founder and developer of the Sacro Occipital Technique (SOT). He graduated from a four-year program in experimental engineering. In 1918 he moved to Detroit to pursue a career in the automobile industry. After an explosion in the factory left him severely crippled, he discovered osteopathy as a possible way to restore his health. He traveled to the Dearborn College of Osteopathy in Elgin, Ill., for treatment. Inspired by his recovery, DeJarnette decided to enroll in the college and was one of four students who studied under the guidance of William G. Sutherland who was largely regarded as the father of cranial osteopathy and one of the principle leaders that helped establish osteopathic craniopathy as a major facet of osteopathy.

After his graduation DeJarnette returned to Lincoln, Neb. Still suffering from serious back problems, he met a chiropractic student who convinced him to receive chiropractic care. After six months of care he was back to normal and decided to enroll in the Nebraska College of Chiropractic, where he received his degree in 1924.

In the 1920s, chiropractic was in its infancy and Dr. DeJarnette with his engineering background and creative mind pieced together one of the first comprehensive approaches to treating the whole body. One of his diagnostic tools involved a muscle testing technique he called mind language. By testing the integrity of a muscle's reflex against the stability of a vertebrae or joint, he could ascertain if a misalignment existed. This diagnostic test become a major part of SOT's comprehensive testing program. One of Dr. DeJarnette's students was Dr. George Goodheart, who broke away from SOT in 1964 to start a new philosophy of chiropractic called Applied Kinesiology.

Applied Kinesiology (AK)

Goodheart challenged old ways, at a time when everyone was using conventional medicines based off of science; Goodheart experimented with new concepts and found that Manual Muscle Testing can pinpoint weaknesses in the body that no other method could. Dr. Goodheart's indefatigable efforts through the 1970s gained him recognition within the health field and he became the first chiropractor to work with American Olympic teams, by serving on the U.S. Olympic Medical team in 1980. Dr. Goodheart's concepts have attracted a dedicated group who have expanded his muscle testing techniques and have established Applied Kinesiology as a major chiropractic philosophy.

Contact Reflex Analysis (CRA)

After graduating in 1959, Dr. Versendaal started his practice in Redlands, California. It was in California that Dick met Dr. Thomas Parker who became his friend and his mentor. Dr. Parker shared his knowledge of nutrition as well as his library of writings by a dentist named Dr. Royal Lee. Dr. Versendaal studied the notes and research finding of this genius doctor and researcher, and applied this knowledge to his own practice. He began to explore the results that could be achieved by matching specific nutrition with specific syndromes. After one year in California, Dr. Versendaal returned to his home in Holland, Michigan. With the seeds of health and nutrition firmly planted, a basic foundation existed for the growth of a new paradigm for health. This was the base upon which Contact Reflex Analysis was developed. The concept and study of reflexes began during the years that Dr. Dick A. Versendaal was attending kinesiology seminars taught by Dr. George Goodheart.

In the 1980s, this author began attending post-graduate courses in nutrition and chiropractic. After taking a Contact Reflex Analysis (CRA) seminar in which I witnessed Dr. Versendaal's technology, I was hooked. I purchased a dozen video tapes of Dr. Versendaal's past seminars. Religiously, I would watch these tapes every weekend until I became familiar with the concepts that Dr. Versendaal researched with the help and combined efforts and expertise of Dr. Peter Northhouse, M.D., Harry Eidenier, Sr., C.N., Dr. Ed Hartman, D.D.S., and Walleed Karachy, a hematologist who correlated the blood and clinical testing to improve its clinical accuracy. These men were invaluable in the research and development of applied clinical nutrition and CRA. This team worked diligently to collect enormous amounts of data, compile, organize, analyze, and to synthesize it into a simple, accurate method that doctors could use in their daily practice. Applying the CRA techniques on my patients open my eyes to the power of natural healing. In 1995, I transitioned into Autonomic Response Testing as developed and taught by Dietrich Klinghardt, MD, PhD and Louisa Williams, DC.

Autonomic Response Testing (ART)

I flew to Seattle, Washington on four separate weekends to study with Dr. Dietrich Klinghardt. His approach opened my eyes to many health issues especially the dental whole body connection. Dietrich's vast knowledge base documented that seventy percent of all medical problems stem from the mouth. It was Dietrich's concepts that enable me to put together the Dental Whole Body Connection seminar series that I use today to enlighten healthcare professionals. It was through his seminars that I was introduced to another genius in the health field, Dr. Yoshiaki Omura, and his concept of Direct Resonance Testing. Fortunately for me Dr. Omura was home based in New York City.

Direct Resonance Testing (DRT)

Studying with Dr. Omura was a real challenge. He was so brilliant that it took me many months to connect the dots he made regarding quantum physics and the frequency connection between the initiators and the disease process. Dr. Omura's patented technology of his testing technique was incredible, clear and precise. As a result of my exposure to these many techniques, I was able to integrate aspects of each one into my Quantum Testing Technique that I routinely use with great success.

The above cliff notes version of the chronological history of the intelligent evolution from simple muscle testing transitioning into the sophisticated Quantum Testing provided me an exciting journey. I had the good fortune of studying with some of the brightest geniuses on this planet. For six years I attended the SOT chiropractic symposiums in Omaha, NE and studied with Dr. DeJarnette and his instructors. He taught me the dental cranial connection, which is an incredible mechanism that has resulted in me being able to resolve numerous chronic pain problems. While attending the SOT meetings, I had the good fortune to meet Dr. Cleo Bludworth, a chiropractor from Ireland, who taught me how to diagnose and correct post-concussion syndrome symptoms that have eluded mainstream medicine. The six years learning SOT manipulative techniques honed my skills and prepared me to handle the difficult clinical cases that come in from all corners of the globe. It is said that there are no accidents. My studying with Drs. DeJarnette, Goodheart, Versendaal, Klinghardt, and Omura was no accident. These professors gave me the pieces to complete the complex puzzle of how the body really works. I was truly humbled by their willingness to share their knowledge. Their dedication to excellence has raised the level of treatment several notches.

Quantum Testing Technique (QTT)

The combined technology of the researchers just mentioned have enabled the formulation of a noninvasive, accurate, cost effective, and expeditious diagnostic and treatment delivery system to solve complex medical issues. Based on quantum physics everything in the universe has a signature frequency at which it vibrates. Dr. Omura utilized and patented this concept as the basis for his diagnostic testing. I refined his approach to make it more user friendly. Genius is simplicity in action. The closer one gets to the truth, the more simplistic the solution.

If a patient has a specific toxin (bacteria, virus, heavy metal, chemical, drug, vaccine and /or adjuvant, etc.), like glyphosate, trapped in an organ or tissue, it can easily be defined as present in the area. By holding a glass pyrex vial that has the actual glyphosate or the frequency of glyphosate in it over the area, if the glyphosate is present, a previously tested strong muscle response will go weak. This is referred to as Direct Resonance Testing. If an organ muscle tests weak, and the patient is then given a vial containing glyphosate to hold in their hand, and the retest tests (indirect testing) strong this is verification that the substance in the vial is present in the organ being tested. If the hand held vial has the exact frequency as that present in the organ being tested, it neutralizes it. This diagnostic approach is capable of pinpointing the presence of toxins in tissues, teeth, jaw bones, brain or anywhere. In contrast, blood tests cannot define the presence of a specific toxin especially if it is trapped within an organ. Blood tests only reflect a reaction to something but does not provide the core reason for the disease.

An example will clarify this concept. A 92-year-old male patient was referred to my office for evaluation and treatment of vertigo that was present for a year and half. Numerous top tier ear nose and throat physicians were consulted during the eighteen-month period with no results. Sir William Osler, the famous Canadian physical stated, "if you listen to the patient long enough, they will give you the diagnosis." The patient repeatedly told all the examining ENT doctors that his vertigo started ten minutes after the drug Ciprodex was applied in his left ear to treat his infection. All the doctors listened but could not interpret what the patient was telling them. When I muscle tested the drug over his left ear, the muscle tested weak signifying the presence of the Ciprodex in the auditory nerve. With a sophisticated electronic device, I made a homeopathic remedy from the actual drug. After applying nine drops of the homeopathic remedy of the Ciprodex in the patient's mouth, his eighteen months of vertigo immediately disappeared and never came back. The beauty about this technology is that it can be applied to any health issue.

Basal Cell Carcinoma

Another case study involving a 62-year-old female patient diagnosed with basal cell carcinoma located on the right side of her nose. The cancer was present for a little over a year. The patient spent several weeks at a notable cancer treatment center in Florida.

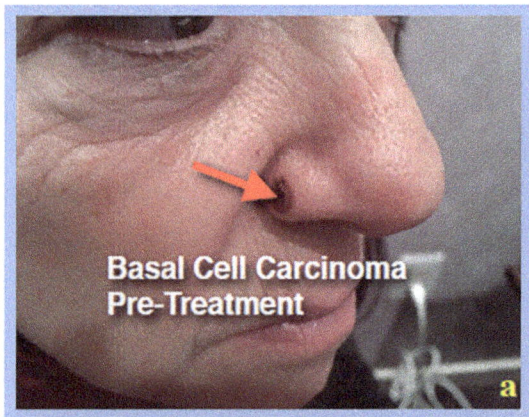

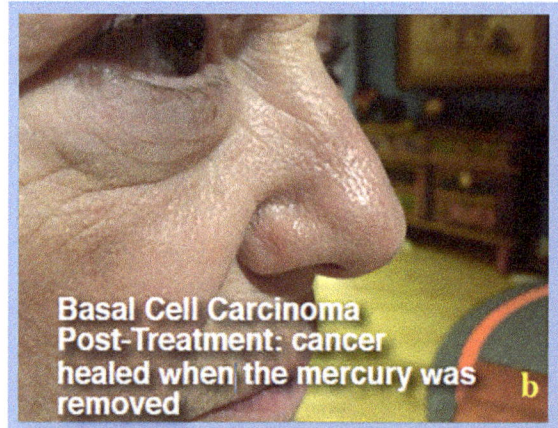

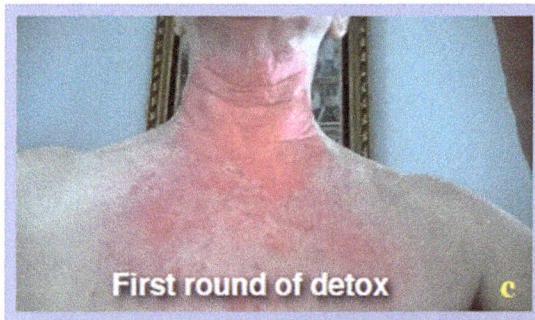

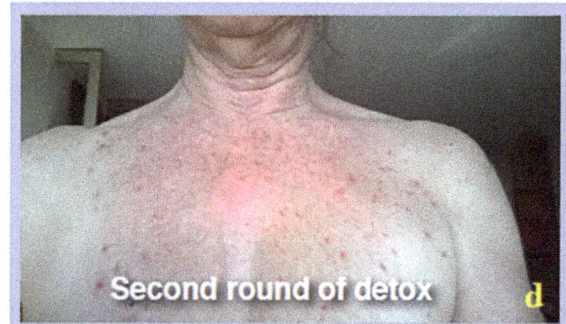

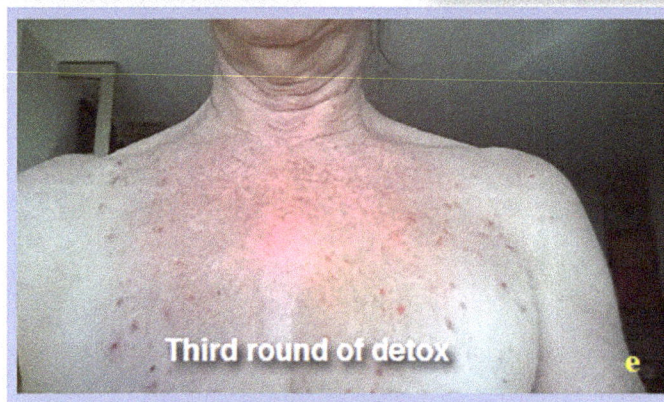

Figures 5 a, b, c, d and e

After a year of wheat grass juice, coffee enemas, acupuncture, dietary and nutritional supplements the cancer was still present. The patient came to my office for consultation.

Examination diagnosed inorganic mercury in the cancerous lesion (Figure 5a). Treatment literally took a year and three months to detox the mercury from the patient. The photographs document the detox reactions from pulling out the mercury plus the cancer disappeared after the "splinter" / initiator was removed. The problem with this approach is that it is too simplistic and mainstream medicine will never buy into it plus they won't be able to charge big bucks for the treatment.

When toxins are expelled from the body, the poisons come out through the various excretory routes: skin, feces, urine, hair, and breath. The severe redness over the patient's thyroid gland (Figure c) denotes that the mercury was concentrated in her thyroid. The patient went through three rounds of detox. At the end of one year and three months the cancer disappeared. Dr. Koch's philosophy about cancer was correct. Cancer is an adaptation and once the initiators are removed the cancer reverts back to healthy cells.

Quantum Testing Technique (QTT)

The Quantum Testing Technique can be used anywhere by anyone who has the skills. One does not require to have expensive computerized equipment to make the diagnosis. Test kits enable the practitioner to quickly define the offending initiators. This concept can even be used to test radiographs. According to my mentor, Dr. Yoshiaki Omura, x-rays of the affected area can be tested the same way as the body is tested. Radiographs, CAT scans, MRIs all capture the frequency of the offending initiators. Often times I use this approach with patients who travel in from foreign countries. This approach expedites my clinical testing by enabling the narrowing down of toxins prior to the patient's visit. By taking this approach it saves office time by focusing in on the causative agents. In addition to testing radiographic records, practitioners can even test the patient's children or pets without them being present. By having the patient write their child's or pet's name on a piece of paper, the practitioner can obtain accurate test result by first testing the owner for pre-existing conditions and then place the paper with the child or pet's name in the owner's pocket. This concept is called quantum entanglement. Everything in the universe is connected energetically.

A case in point. One of my patients asked me to test her friend's dog. Winchester was having daily seizures and the owner's veterinarian could not find the cause with all the blood testing that was done. When my patient was quantum tested with the dog's name in her pocket, mercury showed up in the dog's brain. A liquid homeopathic remedy was prescribed and six weeks later the dog's seizures totally resolved. Winchester has been free of seizures since 2017. This technology is fifty years ahead of what conventional medicine is using. The crime is that they will never embrace these techniques because the pharmaceutical industry, AMA, FDA will never allow it. Change has to come from the consumer. Vote with your pocketbook.

Another interesting case involved a seven-year-old girl who literally was bouncing off the walls. She would not eat, not go to school, and she constantly cried. The child was examined by many medical specialists but no one could make a diagnosis. The little girl would not allow me to even test her so the mother wrote the child's name on a sticky note and placed it in her pocket. I diagnosed hypothyroidism. Because the child would not swallow supplements my technician had to imprint all the vitamins into water. Six weeks later the child's behavior transitioned into normal. This case verifies that it is the frequencies that are doing the healing by resetting the cells function.

Once the "splinters" are defined, the next step is to test which food based nutrients will remove the initiators. Chapter 5 describes this process.

CHAPTER 5

REMEDY SEQUENCING

Setting up a nutritional program can be a daunting process. There are so many antioxidants to choose from and so many so called miracle cancer effective substances. One can spend your children's inheritance if one is not careful. In addition, the choices one has to make regarding various modalities and when to apply them is another arena of confusion. Knowing where to start can be a frustrating experience. I personally went through this process twice. First in 1997 when my wife was diagnosed with breast cancer and again in 2002 when she was diagnosed with stage III ovarian cancer. This section is to take the confusion and fear out of the supplement sequencing procedure.

Watching a professional work in any field always looks easy. The best analogy I can provide is when Michael Angelo, at the age of 29 years-old, was working on his masterpiece, the statue David. An elderly women walked up to him while he was working and commented that it looks easy. Michael Angelo replied to the women "it is lady, you just chip away the pieces you don't want."

The following information was formulated through trial and error over a thirty-five year period. It is based on my own clinical experience of over fifty years of practice as well as input from other professionals with whom I consulted. I realize that one size does not fit all, however, since fifty-four percent of the population has comorbidity issues like diabetes, heart problems and cancer, my approach works in the majority of cases. Like anything else, modifications can easily be made to accommodate variations. Furthermore, finding the right supplements is another major hurdle because not all supplements are of the highest quality. The sequence follows a logical pattern that reduces the incidence of herxheimer's reactions while preparing the body to handle the dumping of toxins. There are six phases of the sequence. Once the rational is learned, chapter six will discuss the specific supplements to consider and test for biocompatibility. Chapter seven will then focus on adjunctive modalities to incorporate to speed the healing process. Chapter eight will focus on integrative medicine. Chapter nine will discuss reconstructing mitochondria, DNA, and healing the body. Chapter ten provides a Nutritional Survival Guide for Cancer and chapter eleven discusses a Comprehensive Approach to Reversing Cancer. Mark Twain said it best, "It ain't what you don't know that gets you in trouble, it's what you know for sure that just ain't so."

The six phases of the nutritional sequence are:

1. Phase I: Detox the liver, intestines, kidney, lymphatics, and restore a healthy microbiome.
2. Phase II: Open up the avenues of excretion.
3. Phase III: Detox the heavy metals.
4. Phase IV: Remove the chemicals especially the herbicide glyphosate.
5. Phase V: Reduce the infections.
6. Phase VI: Remove the vaccines

Phase I deals with cleaning the filter, the liver. The blood of the entire body flows through the liver every three minutes. If the liver cannot pull out and dispose of the toxins through the bile efficiently, then the toxins are recirculated and potentially can get redeposited in various organs and tissues throughout the body.

The thirty feet of our intestines represents 60% to 80% of our immune system. Plus the fact that our intestines have a direct connection to our brain via the lymphatic system and the tenth cranial nerve, the vagus. In my professional opinion, neurodegenerative diseases have been increasing at an alarming rate and I believe one of the main reasons is that our intestines have become extremely toxic due to our environment, poor quality food, water, and air. The intestines must be cleansed, healed, and repopulated with healthy microorganisms. Using special detox formulas will greatly facilitate the cleansing of the liver, lymphatics and kidney.

Phase II focuses on opening up the avenues of excretion. This involves testing nine different homeopathic remedies to ascertain which one best matches the needs of the patient. First, the filter is cleaned then the sewage system must be opened to enable the toxins to leave the cells and travel to the organs of detoxification.

Phase III deals with removing the heavy metals. The most frequently found ones are mercury, cadmium, lead, arsenic, aluminum, and nickel. Interestingly, if the heavy metals are not removed, it is next to impossible to get rid of infections. It appears that the heavy metals impede the function of the immune system. In addition, if the body is deficient in trace minerals (zinc, selenium, manganese, copper, chromium, iodine, indium, molybdenum, iron, and cobalt as part of B12), the body will not let go of the heavy metals. Unfortunately, most people are deficient in trace minerals. A quick check of one's oral pH first thing in the morning will give a good indication of one's mineral reserves. If your oral pH is too acidic (pH below 6.5) then your mineral reserves are low.

Phase IV focuses on the removal of all kinds of chemicals especially the herbicide glyphosate. This toxic herbicide is now ubiquitous in our environment and even found in our rain water; it is also a known carcinogen. Not only does glyphosate cause cancer, it causes leaky gut, leaky brain, primary cause for allergies and general inflammation. Contrary to what the Monsanto executives say it is a poison that will wreak havoc on your body.

Phase V uses special natural antibiotics to reduce the burden of infections. One must be cognizant of the fact that if the body is burdened with a congested liver, toxic intestines, poorly functioning kidneys, slugged up drainage system (lymphatics), heavy metal contamination, chemical toxins, and a weakened immune system (low functioning thyroid and adrenals) and nutritional deficiencies it is virtually impossible to get rid of infections. It is for this reason taking antibiotics to "kill" pathogens is futile and invariably the infections comes back within two weeks after the antibiotics are stopped. The reason why infections exist is because of a polluted terrain and a weakened immune system.

Phase VI deals with the removal of trapped vaccines. This is one area which most conventional and many integrative practitioners are not aware of. The truth is that many patients have childhood vaccines, medications, and toxins trapped in various organs and tissues of the body. How do I know. The following case studies verify this fact.

Case study #1: A patient who was a retired engineer flew in from San Francisco. He presented with a diagnosis of cardiac sarcoidosis (chronic inflammation of the heart). His cardiologist wanted to put him on steroids. He voted with his pocket book and went elsewhere. Interestingly, the Mayo Clinic states on its website that there is no cure for cardiac sarcoidosis and that treatment ranges from steroids to a heart transplant. When questioned about possible exposure to chemicals, he stated that when he grew up in India he and his friends would chase the truck that was spraying DDT. When I tested him with my Quantum Testing Technique he had DDT, glyphosate, cytomegalovirus, and other initiators that were trapped in his heart. Five months later after taking my prescribed supplements to remove the "splinters" the patient returned with a stack of blood tests and a big smile on his face. He stated that all his blood tests were now normal and he had no more heart symptoms.

Case study #2: A patient and her daughter flew in from Iowa. The mother had a diagnosis of systemic lupus a very serious connective tissue disease. The daughter, who was 42 years-old had a right kidney problem since she was five years old. When questioned, the mother gave a history of taking Bendictin during her pregnancy. This drug was used to treat nausea and it is very similar to thalidomide. It was banned in 1985 because of an avalanche of law suites. When examined, the mother had the drug trapped in her liver and the daughter had it trapped in her right kidney. I could not find the drug in the US. I called my friend Peter in Toronto, Ontario whose compounding pharmacist had it in stock. I made a homeopathic from the medication. The daughter's right kidney problem which she had for 37 years disappeared in six weeks. The mother's systemic lupus disappeared in nine months. There is no doubt in my mind about the accuracy of my diagnoses.

Case study #3: Approximately five years ago a patient flew in from Chicago, IL. His chief complaint was that he had internal trembling for a little over one year since he took a prescription of Levaquin (a nasty antibiotic with many side affects). My Quantum Testing Technique verified the presence of Levaquin in his nervous system. I prepared a homeopathic remedy made from the Levaquin. Within 24 hours after taking the homeopathic remedy his internal trembling totally resolved.

Case study #4: I had a patient who was suffering wrist pain for over a year. He was taking Lipitor, a statin drug which causes rhabdomyolysis (breakdown of muscle tissue). A homeopathic remedy was prepared from the Lipitor. After taking the remedy for several days, the patient reported that his wrist pain ceased.

Case study #5: One of my long standing patients, who was a health coach presented with a chief complaint of constant pain in her liver for two weeks. Nothing that she tried had any impact on her pain. Quantum Testing diagnosed the presence of glyphosate in her liver. Instead of preparing a homeopathic remedy, I did a virtual injection. This is a technique I recently pioneered. I tested and determined that the appropriate homeopathic remedy was Iso Pathic Phenolic Rings. I literally pulsed an infrared laser (650 nm) through a pyrex vial that contained the homeopathic remedy into the area of pain. Upon the patient's return visit a week later she reported that by the time she drove home, which was 45 minutes, the pain completely disappeared never to returned. My theory is that the pulsed infrared laser transmitted the frequency of the homeopathic remedy into the area where the glyphosate was trapped and neutralized it. I have had consistent results with other patients that presented similar scenarios with other toxins trapped in their tissues.

Case study #6: A patient, who worked for a pesticide company, was referred to me for evaluation and treatment of Parkinson's disease. The patient walked in flailing his arms and legs all over the place because he had no control. Quantum Testing determined the patient had five pesticides trapped in the left side of his brain. I did a virtual injection with the Iso Pathic Phenolic Rings into his brain on the left side. In addition, he was treated with a scalar energy device, Theraphi, for eighteen minutes. When the patient walked out of the treatment room he was walking almost totally normal. The take-away message in this case is that frequency technology can alter the vibrational pattern of the toxins and neutralize them.

Once an accurate diagnosis is made, the practitioner must have an in-depth knowledge of remedies from which to test. Remedy selection is based on the biocompatibility of the energies of the remedy and the energy pattern of the patient. Remember that less is more. The fewer number of supplements the less chaos created from rapid detox. It is also important to match the energy of the supplement with the energy pattern of the patient. This enhances the healing effect.

Chapter 6 selecting the right remedies discusses an approach that is very accurate and easy to use. Using standard supplement protocols is like throwing darts at the patient. You may get lucky and hit the target once in a while. The Quantum Testing Technique takes the guess work out of the equation.

CHAPTER 6

SELECTING THE RIGHT REMEDIES

Standard Protocol vs Custom

Approaching the treatment of cancer involves defining the "splinters," defining the terrain (tissues too acidic, sympathetic or parasympathetic dominance, hormone imbalances, poor digestion, chronic inflammation, electromagnetic emersion from wi-fi and other EMFs, trapped medications, toxic teeth, etc.), and defining any existing psychological distress factors. Remember distress will lower one's immune system.

Taking a standard protocol of supplements is not a logical path to follow. Remember with no diagnosis there is no treatment. The following listed supplements are those that I test for each of the six phases. Not all of the supplements are used all the time. Only those that test positive. Each must be tested to see if they will work. Every supplement must also be assessed not only for biocompatibility with the patient's energy pattern but also if it will neutralize the specific initiator. My clinical experience has shown that using biocompatible nutrients results in a much better outcome. Can this protocol cure everyone? The answer is emphatically no. There are too many variables to consider and it is virtually impossible to assess them all. In some instances, the immune system is too far damaged from either chemotherapy or the cancer; resurrection of a cancer can be too over whelming for the immune system and therefore it cannot be controlled. In some cases, there are a percentage of people who don't want to live even though they give the impression that they really do. These types can easily be determined by using the person's cranial rhythm. Asking the question subconsciously if they really want to live and then palpitating their cranial rhythm will give you the answer. If the person's cranial rhythm remains symmetrical and balanced when the question is asked, it signifies a yes. If the person's cranial rhythm immediately distorts, then the answer is a no. This is one of the best lie detectors on the planet. I use this technique routinely with all my new patients.

There are literally thousands of supplements to choose from and many different manufacturers offer different formulations. The ones I have chosen are based on my research for the most active ingredients and personal clinical experience. They are by no means the only ones that will bring results.

If the cancer patient is severely ill and toxic, they will have to do coffee enemas to quickly detox the liver. The caffeine in the coffee stimulates the glutathione S-transferase mechanism which allows the liver to quickly dump its toxic burden. The faster the initiators are removed the immune system will become more efficient and the quicker the cells can start to heal. One common denominator in all the major natural cancer therapies is the coffee enema, hold the cream and sugar.

Phase I Supplements: Detox the liver, intestines, kidney, lymphatics, and restore a healthy microbiome.

1. **Glutathione:** Highest concentration is in the liver. It binds to and helps move mercury and other heavy metals out of the tissues and functions as a powerful antioxidant and detoxifier. It protects cells from free radicals and oxidative stress and boosts the immune system. Glutathione's strong antioxidant properties make it suitable in cases of cancerous tumors and lipomas. It also helps the liver detox chemicals and other foreign substances from the blood. It is not able to cure cancer, but several studies suggest that the growth of new cancer cells may be reduced. It also helps protect and reduce the incidence of peripheral neuropathy during chemotherapy with cisplatin drugs.

   Note: I test three different manufacturers of glutathione: Premier Research, Max International, and Quicksilver. There is no one formula that fits all patients.

2. **C3 Curcumin Complex:** Bolsters your immune system, anti-inflammatory, helps regulate digestion, reduces joint and muscle pain, supports brain health and cognitive function, and aids cardiovascular function. Must be taken with a high quality organic, cold pressed oil like sunflower, safflower, or turmeric oil to increase absorption. I use Designs for Health brand.

3. **Cataplex B:** (Standard Process Labs) - Supplies the B-complex vitamins to support liver function. Helps balance the autonomic nervous system by stimulating the sympathetics portion.

4. **Cataplex B2:** (Standard Process Labs) - Supplies the lipotrophic factors for digesting fats; stimulates the parasympathetic part of the autonomic nervous system. Aids the liver in the detoxification process.

5. **Milk Thistle:** Assists in regenerating the liver, promotes bile flow, and is a good antioxidant. I use Energetix brand and Designs for Health brand because the latter has no alcohol. Possible downside of the Energetix brand is that it has 22-28% ethyl alcohol; patients with candida cannot handle the alcohol.

6. **Liver Chi:** It is an all-natural herbal formula to support liver health and detoxification. The herbs in Liver Chi (Bupleurum chinensis, Schizandra chinensis, Smilax glabrahave) have been used for centuries in traditional Chinese medicine as liver tonics and revered for their detoxification properties.

   Available at ICNR, Inc. (www.icnr.com)

7. **Food Grade Diatomaceous Earth:** This product is very effective in killing parasites, absorbing toxins, and scraping the intestinal walls of mucous plaque. Available on Amazon.

8. **Agri-Mectin or IverMectin:** A veterinary product that is safe for humans. Developed by the Japanese and is every effective in killing parasites. Probably the world's most profound anti-viral agent but inexplicably goes unused in the battle against human viral infections, such as COVID-19 coronavirus. Just a single dose of Agri-Mectin abolishes COVID-10

coronavirus in a lab dish. Agri- Mectin works additively with zinc to control viral and bacterial infections.

Dosage: one cc per 100 pounds body weight. Second dose given two weeks later. Available on www.statelinetack.com.

Note: Australia's The Centre for Digestive Disease (CDD) Medical Director Professor Thomas Borody MB, BS, BSc(Med), MD, PhD, DSc, FRACP, FACP, FACG, AGAF, says FDA and TGA approved Ivermectin which he uses regularly in his hospital, has shown positive results for COVID-19.

9. **Serum D$_3$:** It is a pro-hormone. Boosts the immune system, inhibits the replication of cancer cells, and supports the heart. Most cancer patients are deficient. Recommended dosage: 10 drops directly on the tongue upon arising. Contrary to what your physician my say, blood levels for cancer patients should be between 70 - 100 ng/ml. I use Premier Research's Serum D3.

10. **Kaqun Drops:** A liquid probiotic with over 60 different species. Recommend dosage: start with 15 drops in one ounce of spring water upon arising and before bedtime. After two weeks reduce dosage to five drops twice a day. Available from www.icnr.com.

11. **Bravo Probiotic:** One of the best probiotic yogurts on the market especially for cancer patients. It has 42 microorganisms, colostrum, and GcMAF (glycoprotein macrophage activating factor). It also comes in a non-dairy form.

Available at: www.bravo-probiotic-yogurt.com/category/bravo-yogurt

12. **Ph Balancer:** This product is made with non-GMO and organic whole foods, herbs, and extracts. Contains a complete trace mineral profile. Cancer patients invariably are too acidic. An acid pH lowers the oxygen level of tissues and cancer growth is enhanced. If the body is deficient in trace minerals it will not release the heavy metals. Dosage has to be tested. Available from www.Mother Earth Labs.com

13. **Pure Synergy:** This product is made from sixty organic and wildcrafted herbs, grasses, medicinal mushrooms and minerals. It represents living food. Chlorophyll is one of the

best detoxifiers for the body plus supplies vital nutrients for the body to heal. Dosage has to be tested. Available from www.icnr.com.

14. **Clinician's Preference:** Organic, cold pressed formula that provides an 11:1 ratio of omega 6 to omega 3 oils. A vegetable based oil derived from flax oil, evening primrose oil, pumpkin seed oil, and extra virgin coconut oil. Organic, cold pressed Omega 6 oil is anti-inflammatory and helps rebuild the cell membranes. Omega 6 oil acts as a magnet pulling oxygen into the cell. Cancer cannot survive in a highly oxygenated environment. Dosage has to be tested. Available from www.icnr.com.

15. **Indiumease:** Indium is the 49th metal in the periodic table of elements. It opens up all the endocrine organs enabling them to absorb trace minerals. It also is documented to extend one's life. Dosage: three drops directly on the tongue. No food for 10 minutes after taking it. Available from www.icnr.com.

16. **Zymessence:** The best systemic enzyme on the market today. It is anti-inflammatory, antibacterial, mildly antiviral, dissolves foreign protein in the blood and lymphatics, and breaks down the biofilm surrounding cancers. Dosage has to be tested. Available at www. drwongsessentials.com/zymessence/.

17. **Kidney Chi:** It is an all natural herbal formula (Centella asiatica, Lygodium japonicum, Rosa laevigata, Smilax china) that can be used to support kidney and bladder health. Can be combined with Asparagus Extract, an excellent diuretic agent that helps cleanse the kidney. Dosage has to be tested. Available from www.icnr.com.

18. **AMLA -C**: Food based vitamin C made from Indian goose berries. Most vitamin Cs are ascorbic acid which is the antioxidant fraction of vitamin C. Dosage has to be tested. Available at www.icnr.com.

19. **Cordyceps CS4:** It is an adaptogenic mushroom that enables the adrenals to recuperate and function in the resistance stage instead of the exhaustion stage. It is anti-inflammatory, boosts the immune system, increases stamina, and very effective against all forms of cancer. Dosage: three tablespoons per day. Available at www.icnr.com.

20. **Mag O$_7$:** Ozonated form of magnesium that releases O$_2$ breaking down solidified fecal matter in the colon. Removes debris and plaque from intestines and effective against parasites. Dosage: take four capsules before bedtime for one week. If patient is still eliminating chunks at the end of the week, must continue for two or three weeks until all large masses are gone. Available at www.icnr.com.

21. **Liposomal Vitamin C with Lipoic acid:** quenches free radicals, regenerates antioxidants, and alleviates pain. Dosage has to be tested. Available from www.Quicksilver.com.

22. **Superoxide Dismutase (SOD):** SOD is an enzyme found in all living cells. It is essential for liver detoxification. Dosage has to be tested. Available at icnr.com.

The more years I practice the more conservative I become. My mantra is less is more especially when it comes to supplements. Define the "splinters" and define the specific supplements to detox them. You will be amazed how fast the body responds.

23. **Kaqun Water:** Dr. Robert Lyon patented a water that has four molecules of oxygen. Very effective in passing through corrupted cell membranes. One and half liters per day will raise the oxygen content inhibiting growth of cancer cells. Also recommended are 50 minute baths in a more concentrated form. For more information in the USA, please contact Kaqun Wellness Spa Las Vegas - (702) 586-7751. For international locations go to https://kaqun.eu/hungary.

Phase II - Opening up the avenues of excretion

There are nine homeopathic remedies that are tested to determine which one is compatible with the patient. The first four remedies are from Energetix (Atlanta); the second group of five are from Desbio in Utah.

    1.1. **Lymph Tone I:** Lymph drainage (acute)
    1.2. **Lymph Tone II:** Lymph drainage at the cellular level
    1.3. **Lymph Tone III:** Lymph drainage in neoplastic (cancers)

    1.4. **Drainage Tone:** is a homeopathic drainage remedy designed to assist the body in opening blockages within the drainage pathways so toxins can be excreted. Provides gentle yet effective drainage while supporting the immune system.

    1.5. **Lymph Drainage:** Dosage has to be tested.

    1.6. **Kidney Drainage:** Dosage has to be tested.

    1.7. **Liver Drainage:** Dosage has to be tested.

    1.8. **Systemic Drainage:** Dosage has to be tested.

    1.9. **GI Drainage:** Dosage has to be tested.

Use of these homeopathic remedies enhances the drainage of toxins. The faster the poisons can be removed the less of a burden on the immune system.

Phase III: Detox the heavy metals.

Once the liver has been detoxed, trace minerals replenished, microbiome restored, and the avenues of excretion opened, the patient is ready to detox their heavy metals. Bypassing the aforementioned steps will set the patient up for major adverse reactions. If the liver cannot process the heavy metals or other toxins it pulls out from the bloodstream, these poisons recirculate through the body until they get trapped in other organs or tissues and create more inflammation and potential derangement.

There are many nutrients that can be used to chelate out heavy metals. Since 1982, I have tried most of the popular formulas, however, my best results have been with an amino acid product designed by Dr. Bryce Vickery who is the CEO of SuperNutrient. The product is called Platinum Plus. It is gentle and efficient in removing all the heavy metals. Practitioners are cautioned to use a good clay like Clay FX (bentonite or montmorillonite) to adsorb the heavy metals in the gut. It is also imperative to understand that if the heavy metals are not removed it is very difficult to resolve any infections. Also if the body is deficient in trace minerals, it will not let go of the heavy metals. The sequence I have established was formulated after many years of trial and error and has proved to be consistently successful. Each phase is designed to lessen the burden on the immune system, which enhances the body's response to the factors that caused the cancer.

Phase IV: Remove the chemicals especially the herbicide glyphosate.

There is a myriad of nutritional products that are effective in removing chemicals from the body. Like everything else they have to be used and evaluated. The following list comprises those supplements that I have had clinical experience and can validate their effectiveness.

- **Chem Detox (Premier Research):** A unique natural dietary fiber of modified Citrus Pectin that can support the detoxification process and boost immunity.

- **Nutritional Flakes (Premier Research):** This nutritional yeast is a unique, non-GMO vegetarian food with 4 grams of quality protein, containing both essential and non-essential amino acids. This powder is naturally rich in selenium and B-complex to assist the liver in phase II detoxification. It is produced from a specially selected strain of Saccharomyces cerevisiae that is grown on molasses under carefully controlled conditions.

- **Zeolite (Touchstone Essentials):** A natural detoxifier to cleanse the body and digestive system of toxins, heavy metals and pollutants.

- **Glutathione (Premier Research, Max International, and Quicksilver):** Chelates heavy metals, chemicals and supports the immune system.

- **Medi-Chord (Energetix):** Medi-Chord (f.k.a. Chem-Chord) is a homeopathic combination formula for symptoms associated with pharmaceutical or recreational drug usage.

- **Medi-FX Clay (Premier Research):** Medi-Clay-FX™ provides a rare source of calcium bentonite clay that helps promote detoxification. Consuming clay internally has a long history of use with outstanding, health-promoting effects by absorbing intestinal heavy metals and toxins.

- **Detox Balance Program (Standard Process):** provides key nutrients and phytonutrients during all three phases of detoxification that unlock, neutralize, and eliminate toxins. The simple 28-day or 10-day protocol features a tasty, all-in-one detox shake supported by sample meals.

One of the most notorious environmental chemical poisons:

Glyphosate is the most widely used agricultural herbicide in the world, but it's often combined with other toxic herbicides including: Atrazine, 2,4-D (2,4-Dichlorophenoxyacetic acid), Dicamba, and Neonicotinoid insecticides. According to the USDA, more than 225 different pesticides can be found on fruits, vegetables, and grains commonly consumed in the U.S.

Glyphosate is best known as the active ingredient in Roundup-branded herbicides, and the herbicide used with "Roundup Ready" genetically modified organisms (GMOs). Because it's used so heavily, it's now detected in samples of rain water.

Glyphosate binds to minerals (like calcium) and also causes a devastating impact on our internal ecosystem which can result in:

- Deficiencies in essential minerals such as manganese and iron that can lead to diabetes, dementia, and anemia symptoms.
- Overgrowth of pathogens in the gut (dysbiosis or "leaky gut"), which disrupts immune function and increases inflammation, putting you at risk for dozens of chronic diseases.
- Disruption of vital biochemical processes (like detox methylation), which can lead to toxin overload, autoimmune disease and cancer.
- Reduced neurotransmitter production, which can cause depression, anxiety, and cognitive decline.
- Kills off beneficial bacteria (probiotics) while giving dangerous pathogens a competitive edge.
- Creates and speeds up antibiotic resistance in disease-causing bacteria such as salmonella and E. coli.

There are several ways to reduce your body's burden of glyphosate:

- **Citrus pectin:** A soluble fiber known to detoxify heavy metals and clear cholesterol through its superior binding powers.
- **Alginates (purified from kelp):** Proven to protect against pesticide toxicity and effectively remove heavy metals and toxins.

- **Glycine:** An amino acid needed to create glutathione — a powerful detoxifier and antioxidant that also protects the liver against toxicity. Interestingly, the body can mistake glyphosate for glycine during protein synthesis, tricking it into storing toxic glyphosate in tissues and organs. By supplementing with extra glycine, we can prevent glyphosate from being stored, enhance glutathione activity, and help support healthy protein production.

From my research and clinical trials, I have discovered a homeopathic remedy, Iso Pathic Phenolic Rings, from Energetix works incredibly well to remove glyphosate and other pesticides and insecticides. I have even used it in a virtual injection by pulsing a 650nm infrared laser through the homeopathic remedy into the area of the glyphosate. The laser carries the frequency of the remedy into the tissue and neutralizes the glyphosate, insecticide, or pesticide. I discovered this technique when one of my patients who complained of two weeks of constant liver pain was treated with this technique. Forty-five minutes after treatment her two weeks of liver pain disappeared and never came back. I have extrapolated its use to many other situations and it works. Once the burden of the chemicals are reduced, the immune system is stronger and can efficiently deal with infections.

Phase V: Reduce the infections.

When patients have infections, there is a reason. One of the major causes is a weak immune system and from my clinical experience it is often due to a low thyroid; most physicians miss the diagnosis because the blood tests are not accurate. The key to diagnosing hypothyroidism is evaluating the patient's symptom, have the patient take their armpit temperature, and check their pulse. There is a laundry list of symptoms: cold hands and feet, palpitations of the heart, headaches, tinnitus (ring in the ears), dry skin, mental fog, infertility, brittle nails, hair falling out, constipation, depression, anxiety, panic attacks, digestion problems, tooth decay, muscle spasms, ligament weakness, elevated cholesterol, acne, butterfly rash over the bridge of the nose and cheeks, forgetfulness, poor memory, cannot retain what they read, frequent colds/flu, and dizziness. If a patient has a cluster of these symptoms they have a strong probability of having an underactive thyroid. The armpit temperature when taken first thing in the morning before they get out of bed should run between 98.2 ^{0}F and 97.8 ^{0}F. If the temperature runs consistently below 97.8 °F they have a 98% probability of hypothyroidism. The clincher is if their pulse is 72 beats per minutes it confirms the diagnosis. The point to be made is that treating the infections without treating the underlying cause is bad medicine. Unfortunately, most patients and most doctors are looking for the quick fix - antibiotics.

If an underactive thyroid exists, the practitioner must determine what is in the thyroid preventing it from not functioning properly. Whatever is found, it must be removed using food based supplements.

Phase V: Reduce the infections.

It is so much easier to resolve infections once the liver, intestines, kidneys, and lymphatics are cleaned out, and the heavy metals and the chemicals removed. Now the immune system is turbo charged. Whatever remedy is contemplated, it must be tested. Shotgunning is obsolete when you have the diagnostic tools to pinpoint the exact remedy that will work. The following list comprises those natural remedies that work like an antibiotic but do NOT have the adverse side effects:

- **Physician's Strength Oregano**: Very powerful. I resolved a patient in six weeks who had MRSA (Methicillin-Resistant *Staphylococcus Aureus,* which is very contagious. I was the 31st doctor the patient visited. In just six weeks his MRSA was cured.
- **Colostrum (Premier Research)**: Contains proteins called antibodies, which boost the immune system to fight bacteria and viruses.
- **Cordyceps CS4 (ICNR, Inc. USA/ New Me Naturals in Canada):** One of the best supplements to take for cancer or any other illness. It modulates the immune system, it has anti-tumor activity, counteracts fatigue, boosts stamina, boosts the white blood cell count, repairs cells, increases energy, and helps bring the body back to homeostasis or balance.
- **Immutol (Immunocorp):** Oral administration of beta-1,3/1,6-glucans initiate biochemical processes leading to enhanced infection defense, enhanced antibody production against mucosal antigens, enhanced efficacy of injected monoclonal cancer antibodies, faster regeneration of physically damaged tissues, enhanced

healing of (diabetic) wounds, reduced toxicity of bacterial endotoxin, and reduced gut infections.

- **Thymex (Standard Process Labs):** Thymex helps kick-start the thymus gland, the center of the immune system, when antibody production is needed. The thymus is the key immune gland, especially in newborn infants and young children. It preprocesses T-lymphocytes after their origination and migration from bone marrow.
- **Nucleo Immune (Premier Research):** Promotes protein synthesis, cellular vitality, beneficial intestinal flora and immune system health. Nucleotides function as cellular signaling molecule.
- **Noni (Premier Research):** According to the National Centre for Complementary and Integrative Health, noni juice has tumor fighting and immune stimulating properties. Prevents cancer and boosts immunity. Noni fruit is rich in antioxidants, Vitamin C, Vitamin B3, Vitamin A and Iron. Noni juice is said to be a magical drink as it affects so many bodily systems positively.

The key points to walk away with are first define the infecting agent and second define which nutrients will counteract the pathogens. This approach is logical, cost effective, and accurate. Physicians have to stop throwing medical darts and start focusing on the core issues.

Phase VI: Remove the vaccines

In my thirty-five-year quest to find the best sequence, I found that removing childhood or any vaccines was the most difficult. The lightbulb finally went on after completing all the five Phases of detox. I finally realized that the cleaner the body the more efficient the detox mechanism and the easier it was to remove the vaccines. Contrary to what your family physician thinks, vaccines like other chemical drugs have the potential to get trapped within organs or tissues. Conventional blood test will not find these hidden culprits. Only by using energetic testing, Quantum Testing Technique or similar method, can they be discovered.

Following the principle rules I established, the first item is to identify the trapped vaccine. Second rule is to test the homeopathic nosode potency required to neutralize it and third is to establish the dosage (how many pellets or drops) and best time to take the remedy. 'Nosode' is the term used for a specific group of remedies widely used in homeopathic prescribing. Nosodes are made from disease products of human or animal origin and they have been an essential part of the European homeopathic tradition for over two hundred years. Results from clinical trials and data collection in homeopathic practice show a long track record of safety for these products.

Many of the homeopathic nosode remedies have to be custom made. I have been using a company, Celletech in Madison, Wisconsin for years with great success. If your naturopathic doctor or other professional practitioner is interested they can be reached at (800) 888-4066.

Homeopathy has been under attack by the established pharmaceutical cartels for being bogus. My response is simple. If homeopathy is so fraudulent, why did the royal family of England use a homeopathic physician, Peter Fisher for seventeen years, to prescribe homeopathic remedies? It is also reported that when the Queen travelled abroad she always took her leather case containing her homeopathic remedies. The real reason for the attack is that homeopathy is too effective and much less expensive than drugs and there are little or no side effects.

CHAPTER 7

ADJUNCTIVE MODALITIES IN CANCER TREATMENT

The New Millennium has ushered in a major paradigm shift in medicine: define and treat the underlying cause. Based on concepts of quantum physics and integration of many specialties, this unique therapy is called Quantum Medicine. Based on intelligent evolution, patented technologies, and outside the box innovative thinking a more comprehensive evaluation and treatment approach now exists. Enlightened practitioners can now look at the patient globally and incorporate factors which traditional medicine reject, discount or are not even aware.

Truth About Laboratory Testing

Traditional laboratory blood tests only reveal reactions to dysfunction but they do not define the underlying cause. From this perspective, traditional blood testing is obsolete. This diagnostic vacuum was filled with computerized programs that use a holographic energy pattern of the patient to compare known frequencies of heavy metals, viruses, bacteria, chemicals, vaccines, hormones, etc. From this comparison, a computer analysis can produce a list of the primary stressors in the body. One such energy device is called CyberScan System.

CyberScan Professional System

During the past 25 years patients have witnessed incredible advances in medical technology which have improved their quality of life. As a result of this intelligent evolution, the CyberScan Professional System evolved. This system has incorporated the genius of Nicola Tesla's discovery of scalar waves and the most advanced concepts of Quantum Physics. The benefits of this integration is that health problems can now be solved quicker and more cost effectively. By using non-invasive scalar wave technology practitioners can now correct abnormal energy fields surrounding cells. When the morphogenic or energy field around the cell becomes normalized it communicates this information to the internal parts and reprograms the cell to work normally. When cells function normally the symptoms disappear.

The CyberScan System approaches health issues in several ways. First phase detects the underlying stressors initiating your problem. The underlying stressors are corrected during the first three-month treatment period. Most patients baseline energy pattern is re-evaluated every two weeks. If your health issues are more serious, you may require more attention on a weekly basis. CyberScan also addresses EMFs (Electromagnetic Frequencies), wi-fi, cell phone frequencies and much more. A custom eeCard is also specifically programed to meet your EMF needs. By placing this card under your mattress where your feet lie, while you sleep, it protects against potentially dangerous EMF frequencies. This "insurance" policy helps you obtain a more restful night's sleep. One can imprint the healing frequencies from the eeCard, directly into your bottled spring water. By placing the bottle of water directly on top of the magnetic strip of the card there is a transfer of the scalar waves and healing frequencies into the water, which is a crystal and can hold the frequencies. Drinking the water places the healing frequencies in your system for more effective results. A new eeCard is made with each new analysis during the one to two-week interval between visits. Phase two focuses on regeneration during the second three-month period. Once the offending factors are removed the scalar waves start the restoration of normal healthy function.

Melanoma Diagnosed by CyberScan Professional System

A 58-year-old female patient was evaluated with the CyberScan System. The patient presented with a multitude of health issues. One of the key findings in the CyberScan Report was the presence of melanoma on the skin. When the patient returned home to Florida she made an appointment with her dermatologist. The physician's thorough examination located the melanoma and surgically removed the lesion. Traditional testing doesn't come close to the accuracy and noninvasiveness of the CyberScan System.

I have used this system in my practice since 2012 with incredible results. CyberScan quickly scans the morphogenetic or energy fields around cells, determines where the stressors are within the body, and creates a 100% natural scalar information carrier that communicates, as well as stimulates, the self-healing properties of the immune system. The CyberScan System also has the capability to broadcast the healing frequencies to patients any where in the world. Scalar waves travel multiple times faster than the speed of light contrary to what Albert Einstein told us. This characteristic enables the scalar waveform to reach the patient in nanoseconds. Because the original scan captures the holographic pattern of the patient it also captures their DNA signature. When the scalar waves are sent out, they will only be attracted to the individual that matches the DNA pattern. This is similar to a TV station broadcasting its signals of a particular show. If your set is tuned to that specific frequency, it will pick up that show.

Nikola Tesla's Scalar Energy Can Restore Cellular Integrity or More Simply Put Restore Your Body Back to Factory Default

Theraphi Plasma System—Intelligent Evolution

Did you ever wish you could turn back your physiologic clock? This wishful thinking is now a reality. It's called Theraphi Plasma System. This incredible technology uses scalar energy to restore your body back to a state when it was healthy. It sounds too good to be true, but in this case it really is true. The benefits of scalar energy have been known since the 1960's when Antoine Prioré, an Italian researcher, working in France discovered the healing powers of scalar energy. Why hasn't the medical reporter on the 11' o' clock news mentioned it? The answer is simple. Scalar energy devices reduce the profits of the pharmaceutical cartel. By the end of the 1970's Antoine Prioré was healing almost 100% of all types of cancers and diseases. Then the research funds abruptly stopped.

Scalar energy provides the template to heal the body's DNA. Its spiral double-helix waveform is the same as DNA and the most efficient pattern for growth and repair. This unique energy pattern also has the ability to bring together raw materials in your body and make what it needs for the repair process. In reality, scalar energy is the "Holy Grail" of healing. Scalar energy's creative forces enable it to disassemble the energy pattern of toxins, viruses, bacteria, fungi, parasites, chemicals, vaccines as well as any other foreign matter that interferes with your health. It is also the carrier wave for human emotion as well as the body's memory system. It's like the hard drive in your computer. It stores the files which make your body function.

Scalar energy is the Life Force of the universe and our body. In the 1940s, this was proven by Thomas Galen Hieronymus, an engineer genius, who grew healthy plants in total darkness. Hieronymus discovered that it was the scalar energy, not the electromagnetic waveform of light, that stimulates photosynthesis. Scalar energy is produced by the sun. This is why the ancients worshiped the sun god. They had good reason.

How effective is scalar energy clinically? In my 50 plus years of clinical practice, I have come to the conclusion that the common denominator for achieving real healing and health is with the use of frequencies. The Theraphi Plasma System, which is now available in my practice, utilizes 18 specific healing frequencies coupled with a Bio-Active Plasma field of scalar energy to affect cellular regeneration. A treatment session can vary from 3 to 18 minutes and is totally non-invasive with only positive side effects.

A recent patient came in with low back pain of several weeks duration. The pain was due to a rear-end collision. Five minutes of exposure to the scalar energy produced by the Theraphi Plasma System totally resolved her pain.

Five Months of Left Knee Pain Resolved in Two Days with Theraphi

An example of Theraphi's incredible effectiveness was recently witnessed when one of my patients who experienced left knee pain since March 2016 had total resolution in two days with just two five minutes sessions. He had sought acupuncture, chiropractic and massage therapy during the five-month period with no lasting results. Of interest, a decrease in the inflammatory process was documented by means of infrared photography. A dramatic decrease of 11.54°F drops in temperature occurred immediately following treatment on the second day. The patient was in awe of the results.

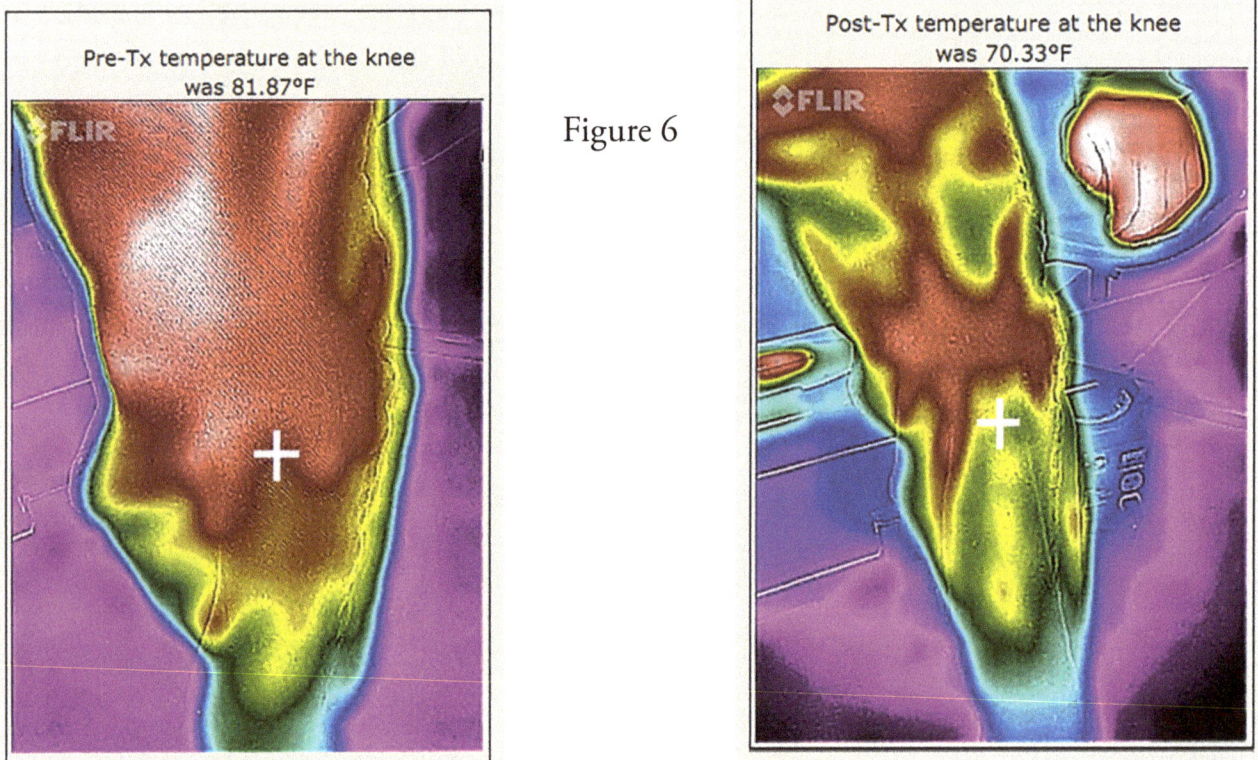

Figure 6

Someone once said that the closer you get to the truth the more simplistic the solution. This certainly is the case for the Theraphi Plasma System.

The Theraphi Plasma System integrates the research of Royal Raymond Rife's healing frequencies from the 1930's, Nikola Tesla's noninvasive scalar wave electrotherapy from the 1920's, Antoine Prioré's electromagnetic healing technology from the 1960's and '70's, and Georges Lakhovsky, a Russian physicist, who in 1925, while living in France, integrated the research of the three aforementioned pioneers. The ultimate benefit of the plasma generator is that the coherent electromagnetic field created by the Theraphi System restores your body to its original condition. In other words, your cells revert back to a factory default setting when everything was in a state of health. This represents anti-aging at its finest.

The work of Vlail Kaznacheyev, a Russian researcher in the mid-1970's showed that use of scalar electromagnetic waves can reverse cell death and the disease process. Rife, Prioré, Lakhovsky, and Kaznacheyev successfully reversed cancers in animals and Rife in humans. By reversing the aging process this technology has been shown to be effective for:

- Pain reduction
- Reduction of inflammation
- Tissue regeneration
- Enhancing cancer remission
- Anti-aging
- Cell memory reversal
- Reversing cancer

It becomes an obvious conclusion that if a cell that is in a pathological, abnormal or diseased state can be reversed, then diseases such as MRSA, Alzheimer's, dementia, heart disease, sports and other types of injuries and other medical illnesses can also be reversed.

Innovative Technology Using Hyperpolarized Light to Heal the Body

Quantum Healing with Hyperpolarized Sunglasses

The use of light for healing is not a new concept. However, the use of hyperpolarized sunglasses as a new healing modality provides healthcare practitioners with an innovative technology that has great healing potential. The Swiss company, Zepter, has pioneered the use of man-made full-spectrum light for enhancing the body's ability to restore homeostasis. A recent clinical observation has spawned a new paradigm for patient treatment.

Since the human body functions within a normal frequency ranging from 62 to 68 MHz, any alteration that lowers the frequency range transitions the body into the disease process. It has been documented that disease starts at 58 MHz with the appearance of colds and flu at 57 to 60 MHz, Epstein Barr virus occurs at 55 MHz, cancer initiates at 42 MHz, and death starts at 25 MHz. Elevating the body's frequency level by means of raw organic foods, homeopathic remedies, food based vitamins, minerals, scalar waves, essential oils, prayer and meditation, music, sunlight, Rife frequencies, and color light therapy all function to restore health.

In the 1970s, a German researcher by the name of Fritz Albert Popp discovered that carcinogens, like mercury, prevent the body from absorbing the wavelength of 380 nm to repair the DNA. This process triggers degeneration and disease. This blocking effect holds true for all carcinogens and prevents the DNA repair process.

Fortuitously, this researcher recently discovered that placing the Tesla Lightwear glasses on someone who had a toxic substance like mercury in their pocket negates the deleterious effect of the mercury. The subject was tested kinesiologically to establish a baseline muscle response. The muscles tested strong. Then a vial of mercury was placed in the subject's pocket, and they were retested. The retest resulted in the subject not being able to hold up their arms. The Tesla Lightwear glasses were then placed over their eyes while the vial of mercury was still in their pocket, and the subject tested stronger than had been on the baseline test. My hypothesis is that the frequency generated by the vial of mercury disrupted the subject's energetic field. Placement of the Tesla Lightwear glasses stimulated the central and peripheral nervous systems, via the optic nerve, with full-spectrum light (430–770 THz - minus the infrared and blue portions) to raise the energy field of the entire body from the inside outward. I believe this higher frequency has the beneficial effect of negating the 13 to 21 toxic frequencies that mercury produces. Extrapolating this finding, my theory is that wearing the Tesla Lightwear glasses will neutralize all toxic energy fields from pesticides, chemicals, heavy metals, vaccines, viruses, etc. by raising the frequency level of the body's energy field. In essence, the full-spectrum light will either transmutate toxic energy fields into nontoxic energy or erase them. Further study is needed to confirm these observations.

Quantum Healing with the Bioptron Full-Spectrum Light Therapy System

Full spectrum light research started in 1903 with a Nobel Prize in Physiology, awarded to Niels Ryberg Finsen for his use of concentrated ultraviolet light to treat Lupus vulgaris, a form of tuberculosis (TB) that attacks the skin. Since then, light research has continued at an unprecedented pace. For decades the different effects of the colors have been observed, studied and recorded. Hospitals have successfully used blue light for infants with jaundice and red light for tuberculosis. Today NASA, is using the far infrared light (670nm wave length) as a stand-alone therapy for plant growth to stimulate natural cell energy and for wound healing for astronauts. One of the main reasons why the Bioptron System with its full spectrum light therapy is so effective is because it increases circulation by 48%, which increases oxygen absorption, stimulates nerve function and enhances and regulates immune function. An example of the powerful healing benefits of the Bioptron System is seen in a case of basal cell carcinoma. The Bioptron was applied to the basal cell carcinoma for twenty minutes twice a day for three weeks. The increased circulation of blood, increased oxygen absorption, and accelerated production of adenosine triphospate (ATP - molecule that stores energy) literally healed the tissue beneath the cancer forcing it out of the body. In essence, it represents nature's own microsurgery system.

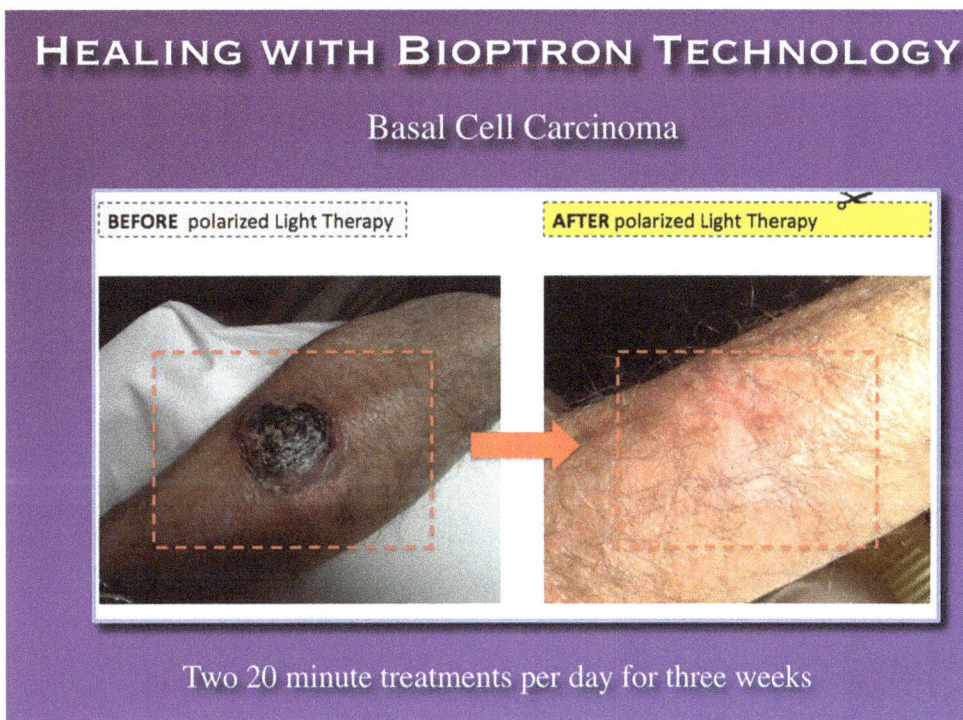

HEALING WITH BIOPTRON TECHNOLOGY

Basal Cell Carcinoma

BEFORE polarized Light Therapy · AFTER polarized Light Therapy

Two 20 minute treatments per day for three weeks

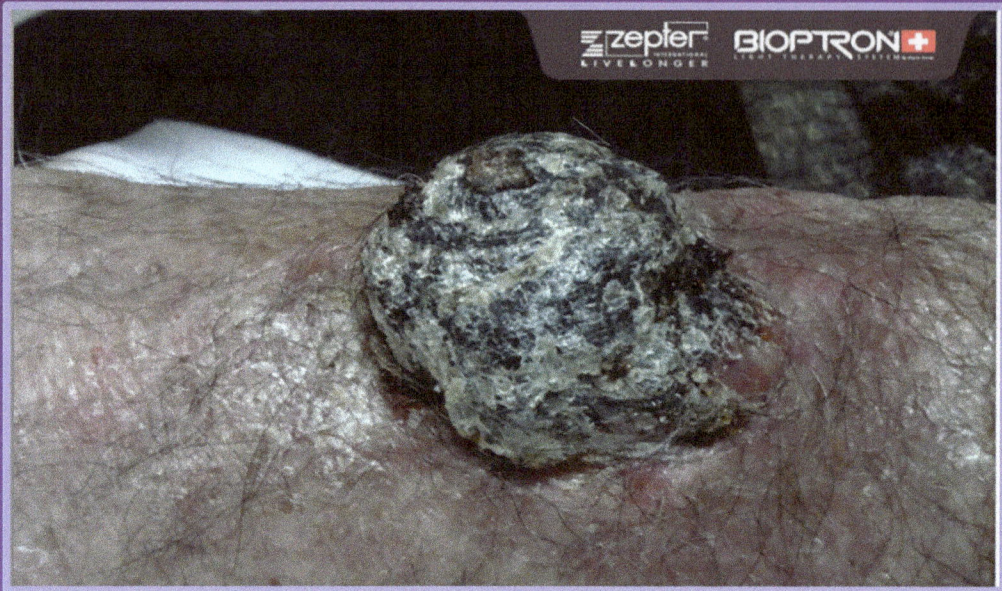

HEALING WITH BIOPTRON TECHNOLOGY
Basal Cell Carcinoma

ANSAR Medical Technology Testing: Evaluates both the Parasympathetic & Sympathetic Nervous System Function

ANSAR testing represents one area in medicine that is often overlooked because practitioners are unaware of the latest FDA approved technology. Simply put, the ANSAR testing system is a painless, non-invasive diagnostic procedure that determines how well a patient's autonomic nervous system is functioning.

The autonomic nervous system is the involuntary part of everyone's neurological make-up and manages just about every system in the body. It controls digestion, sleep, breathing, circulation, blood pressure, heart rate, even stress. The list is practically endless.

The autonomic nervous system is divided into two parts: the parasympathetic and the sympathetic.

The parasympathetic half handles normal conditions, such as digestion, healing, blood flow and respiration.

The sympathetic part of the nervous system controls the body's reactions during times of illness, stress or injury. It prepares the body to react (the "fight or flight" response). Heart rate increases as does blood pressure and respiration. The body is directed to release glucose, adrenaline and other stress hormones.

In a perfect world, the autonomic nervous system maintains its balance. This is not always the case. When there is an imbalance, there is a reason. ANSAR testing can detect many conditions in the early stages, when treatment can be most effective. Cardiovascular disease, diabetes, Parkinson's disease, multiple sclerosis, chronic fatigue syndrome and high blood pressure are just some of the conditions that can be identified and measured with the ANSAR test.

ANSAR testing provides practicing physicians with very detailed and specific data. This is a customized approach to medicine. The diagnosis and treatment for one patient will differ from that of another based on the information from the ANSAR test. In addition, follow up testing can objectively document if the treatment provided is making the patient better or worse. This technology raises the level of excellence and should be a part of every practice.

One of the principal issues with today's medicine is that the majority of the diagnostic tests do not uncover the underlying causes of the patient's illness. One solution to this problem is the use of a software program developed by MIT and integrated into a computer system, ANSAR, that can analyze the autonomic nervous system. It has been recognized by many medical authorities that an imbalance of the autonomic nervous system is the reason for many dysfunctions of the body.

An example of such an imbalance was recently uncovered when one of my patients presented with chief complaints of fatigue and mental fog especially after lunch. None of the conventional medical testing uncovered the cause of the patient's complaints. Evaluation by the ANSAR (autonomic nervous system analysis report) testing showed that the patient's parasympathetic (similar to the breaks in a car) and the sympathetic (similar to the gas pedal in a car) were both low. Rather than prescribing drugs for the symptoms, nutritional supplements were provided to correct the underlying problem rather than mask it. The patient's problems completely resolved.

The advantages of the ANSAR system is that it records both the parasympathetic and sympathetic parts of the nervous system whereas most heart rate monitoring systems on the market only evaluate the sympathetic portion. The result is a much more comprehensive examination and a more valid assessment of the patient. Preclinical issues like the potential for sudden cardiac death, hypotension and hypertension issues can be determined before they manifest into clinical symptoms.

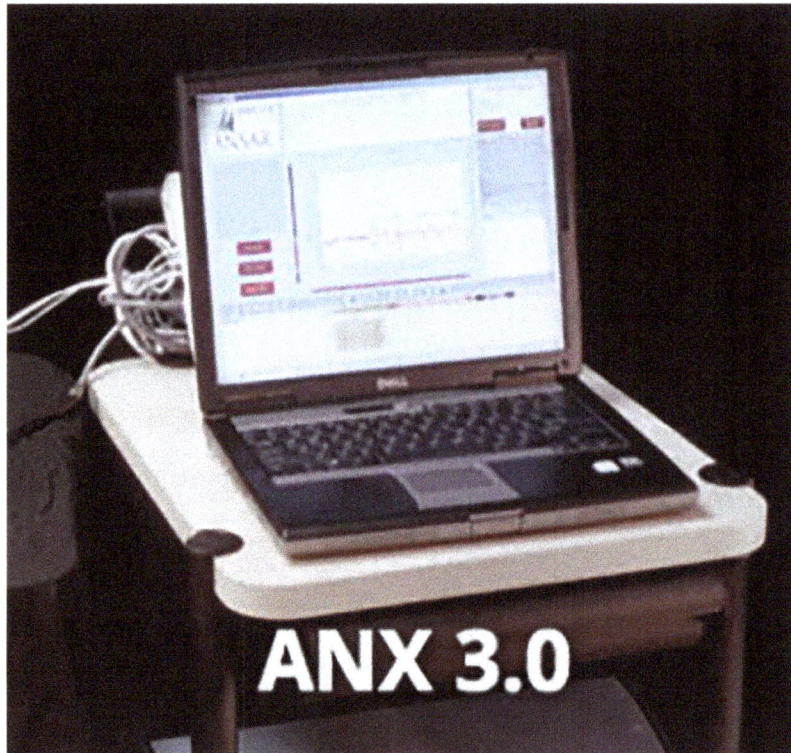

In a cliff notes description, the ANSAR system evaluates by means of an EKG reading of the patient in six parameters: baseline resting, deep breathing (parasympathetic assessment), baseline resting, Valsalva (short rapid breaths assessing the sympathetics), baseline resting, and standing (assessing the sympathetic nervous system). By assessing these various parameters a noninvasive comprehensive evaluation of the patient is obtained.

Most medical practices and even cardiologists do not offer this type of comprehensive evaluation.

Available from **Physio PS, Inc. ;** 86 Nashua Rd, Londonderry, NH, 03053 (603) 320-0836; for information contact Steve O'Leary: soleary@physiops.com

Ozone: One of the Miracle Cures for Cancer

Ozone therapy has been in use since Nikola Tesla patented his ozone generator in 1896. Ozone is incredibly effective for the treatment of viruses, bacteria, candida, fungi, parasites, yeast, cancer, and all types of toxins. It literally destroys pathogens and toxins on contact making them water soluble and easily excreted.

Once one understands the nature of cancer one can easily understand why ozone therapy is so effective. Traditional medicine keeps disseminating the myth that there are 100 plus different types of cancer and that is why radiation, surgery and the different types of chemotherapy drugs are needed. The truth is that **ALL CANCERS** are the same. Cancer is an adaptation to environmental toxicity. One of the key factors in the cause of cancer is hypoxia or low oxygen. This results from the cell membranes becoming corrupted from adulterated omega 6 oils (safflower, sunflower, canola, corn, soy, cottonseed, walnut), all of which are pro-inflammatory. When these adulterated oils become incorporated into the cell membrane, it literally turns it to plastic. A plastic membrane impedes the entrance of oxygen and nutrients and the exiting of metabolic wastes. The end result is hypoxia. Deprivation of oxygen to the cells resulting from air pollution, processed and adulterated foods, chemically polluted water, and a sedentary lifestyle encourages anaerobic (low oxygen environment) microbes to proliferate. Over-growth of harmful pathogens will lead to breakdown of enzymatic reactions, overload of metabolic wastes and ultimately cell death.

Under anaerobic (low oxygen) conditions, cells will mutate to a more primitive life form, transitioning from aerobic (air) to anaerobic (no air) respiration for energy synthesis. Nobel prize winner Dr. Otto Warburg won a Nobel Prize in Physiology in 1931 because he documented that the primary cause of cancer is the replacement of oxygen in the respiratory chemistry of normal cells by the fermentation of sugar. The growth of cancer cells is a fermentation process which can be initiated only when the oxygen level drops by 35 percent. Ozone being a gas can easily pass through the corrupted cell membrane and it produces short-lived peroxides. Cancer cells lack the enzyme glutathione peroxidase to counteract the peroxides and that is why they cannot survive in a highly oxygenated environment. It is recommended that vitamin E, N-acetyl-cysteine, and selenium be administered during ozone therapy to support the glutathione detoxification system. In addition, a mixture of an 11:1 ratio of organic, cold pressed omega 6 to omega3 oils be supplied. Organic, cold pressed omega 6 oils help repair the cell membrane and are anti-inflammatory, and act as a magnet pulling the oxygen into the cells. This is a key factor that is missing in most cancer treatment protocols.

Ozone Activates Immune System

The medical literature documents ozone's ability to activate macrocytes, monocytes, and lymphocytes and stimulate the production of cytokines such as interleukin, interferon, and tumor-necrosis factor (The Journal of International Medical Research 1994). Its ability to elicit endogenous production of cytokines and its lack of toxicity make ozone an indispensable therapeutic modality especially since most devastating diseases, viral diseases, cancer and AIDS, are characterized by a depressed immune system.

Today ozone is used to enhance the body by:

- Stimulating the immune system to speed up healing (SARS, Ebola, MRSA, AIDS)
- Improving circulation by cleaning the arteries and veins (reduce plaque build-up)
- Purifying blood and the lymph of foreign protein and debris
- Normalizing hormone and enzyme production
- Having anti-inflammatory properties
- Reducing pain (injection into joints, muscles, etc.)
- Stopping bleeding
- Prevents shock
- Limiting stroke damage
- Reducing cardiac arrhythmia or abnormal heart rhythm
- Reducing the risk of complications from diabetes
- Improving brain function and memory

The real problem with ozone is that it is relatively inexpensive, too effective and offends Big Pharma by reducing their profits.

Case Studies

The following case summaries are just some examples of ozone's effectiveness.

Case # 1: Ninety-two year-old caucasian male diagnosed with liver cancer. In just five treatments the patient stopped rectal bleeding, increased his sense of well-being and mental clarity and his energy soared.

Case # 2: Forty-five-year-old female presented with an upper respiratory infection. Three ozone therapy sessions via ear insufflation resolved her sneezing, fever, and coughing.

Case #3: Seventy-five-year-old male presented with benign enlarged prostate, frequent and impeded urination. Six ozone treatments resolved the symptoms.

If you're interested in learning more about which ozone system I recommend you go to <u>www.icnr.com/articles/ozone-use-in-healing.html</u>.

Advantages of Homeopathic Remedies in Cancer Therapy

Homeopathy is more than 200 years old. It is one of the most common complementary therapies used by people with cancer. Homeopathy is based on the theory of 'like cures like' and the 'law of the smallest dose.'

When properly used, homeopathic remedies offer individuals:

- Non-invasive approach
- Non toxic to the patient
- Means of curing the underlying problem
- Cost effective treatment
- Quicker recovery period
- Reduced risk of adverse side effects

No matter what combination of symptoms or chief complaints the individual is suffering at any given time they are all manifestations of a single "disease" that is unique to that individual. The homeopathic philosophy believes that no one organ of the body can be ill without affecting the person as a whole. All symptoms, therefore, must be analyzed and taken into account since they all represent the body's effort to heal itself. Individuals who present recurrent acute or chronic episodes of an illness are reflecting a "constitutional" weakness. The goal of homeopathy is NOT to treat the symptoms but use them as a guide for the appropriate remedy that will stimulate the person's defense system.

The remedy Carcinosin is often used successfully in the treatment of Cancer. Carcinosin is made by first preparing a specimen of the cancerous tissue, usually taken from the breast, and subsequently sterilizing and dissolving it in disinfected water. This blend is then diluted as well as succussed repeatedly; the remedy is tapped against one's palm to "imprint" the energetic force of the remedy into the molecular structure of the liquid.

While we are uncertain who was the first to use cancer nosodes we know that Dr. J.C. Burnett was the first person to write about their use. Dr. Burnett also proved this remedy on himself and the symptoms that they produced in him were that he felt a deathly sinking, sickly sensation.

J. Clarke records many cases where he successfully used the cancer nosode to cure cancer, Carcinosin being the most predominant. He says; "Of all the remedies for cancer, in my experience the cancer nosodes form the most important class and the use of them ought to be more familiar to homoeopaths themselves".

Cooper also relates numerous cases in which he has successfully used Carcinosinum 200 and states; "I would lay it down as a maxim that there is no case of carcinoma that Carcinosinum would not benefit from at some period of its existence, so much so that I would suggest the proverb; 'When in doubt give Carcinosinum.'

A.U. Ramakrishnan, MD has been using cancer nosodes in cancer treatment for the last thirty years and he is leading the world in the homoeopathic treatment of cancer, treating at least 2000 cancer patients a year. One of the nosodes he uses is Carcinosinum.

An advantage of this remedy was that Carcinosinum can relieve cancer pains. Carcinosinum won't cure cancer, but according to James Tyler Kent, MD, the forefather of American homeopathy, it will palliate the cancer for years taking away the sharp, burning and tearing pains.

The homeopathic remedy Ruta graveolens 6 selectively induces cell death in brain cancer cells but proliferation in normal peripheral blood lymphocytes: A novel treatment for human brain cancer

INTERNATIONAL JOURNAL OF ONCOLOGY 23: 975-982, 2003

SEN PATHAK1,2, ASHA S. MULTANI1, PRATIP BANERJI3 and PRASANTA BANERJI3

Departments of 1 Cancer Biology and 2 Laboratory Medicine, The University of Texas M.D. Anderson Cancer Center, Houston, TX 77030, USA; 3 PBH Research Foundation, 10/3/1 Elgin Road, Kolkata 700 020, West Bengal, India - Received April 16, 2003; Accepted May 28, 2003

Abstract.

Although conventional chemotherapies are used to treat patients with malignancies, damage to normal cells is problematic. Blood-forming bone marrow cells are the most adversely affected. It is therefore necessary to find alternative agents that can kill cancer cells but have minimal effects on normal cells. We investigated the brain cancer cell-killing activity of a homeopathic medicine, Ruta, isolated from a plant, Ruta graveolens. We treated human brain cancer and HL-60 leukemia cells, normal B-lymphoid cells, and murine melanoma cells in vitro with different concentrations of Ruta in combination with tricalcium phosphate ($Ca_3(PO4)_2$. Fifteen patients diagnosed with intracranial tumors were treated with Ruta 6 and $Ca_3(PO4)_2$. Of these 15 patients, 6 of the 7 glioma patients showed complete regression of tumors. Normal human blood lymphocytes, B-lymphoid cells, and brain cancer cells treated with Ruta in vitro were examined for telomere dynamics, mitotic catastrophe, and apoptosis to understand the possible mechanism of cell-killing, using conventional and molecular cytogenetic techniques. Both in vivo and in vitro results showed induction of survival-signaling pathways in normal lymphocytes and induction of death-signaling pathways in brain cancer cells. Cancer cell death was initiated by telomere (protect individual chromosomes) erosion and completed through mitotic catastrophe events. We propose that Ruta in combination with $Ca_3(PO4)_2$ could be used for effective treatment of brain cancers, particularly glioma blastoma.

Summary

In contrast to conventional chemotherapy that kills not only cancer cells but also normal cells, the Ruta 6 + Ca3 (PO4)2 combination kills glioma brain cancer cells selectively and protects normal lymphocytes by inducing cell division in blood-forming cells. This homeopathic medicine could be prescribed for optimum treatment of brain cancers in general, and gliomas in particular, as well as possibly reducing severe side effects and protecting blood-forming cells in these patients.

The walk away message is that there are no magic bullets, however, when homeopathics are combined with a comprehensive approach of defining the underlying cause(s), detoxing the body by removing the heavy metals, chemicals, vaccines, herbicides, etc., supplying real organic foods and food based supplements geared to the removal of the "splinter," patients have the best chance of reversing the cancer.

Removing Vaccines with Homeopathic Nosodes

One main stressor that faces patients and especially cancer patients is the presence of trapped vaccines: both childhood and any vaccination thereafter. Conventional medicine does not know that they do not know that vaccines can become trapped within organs and tissues. When present they offer an interference field to the body and cause stimulation to the adrenal glands. The internationally known researcher, Han Selye, MD, documented in his 1936 research that the adrenal glands respond the same way to physical, chemical, and psychological distress. Phase six addresses the vaccine issue. Homeopathic nosodes are used to discharge the trapped vaccine that has been imbedded in tissues. The following clinical photograph documents the detox reaction that occurred when a vaccine nosode was use to remove childhood vaccines that were trapped in the patient's abdomen.

Vaccine Detox Reaction

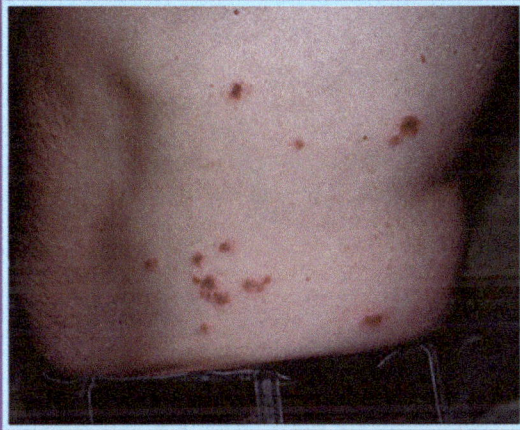

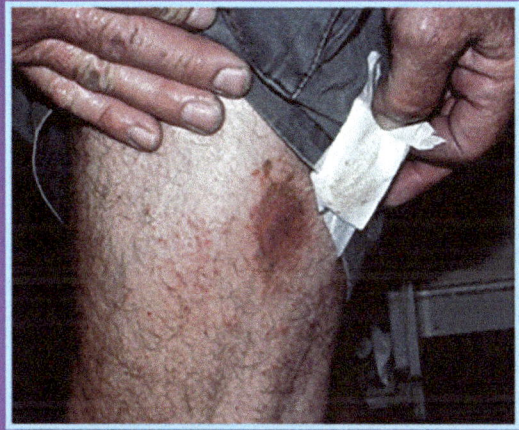

Use of homeopathic nosodes to remove old childhood vaccinations can cause an adverse detoxification reaction if you do not prepare the body to handle the detox.

The treating physician's primary goal should be, preparing the body to handle the dumping of toxins, opening up the avenues of excretion, removing the heavy metals, herbicides, pesticides, insecticides, and any trapped vaccines. This approach should also be complemented with adjunctive therapies to enhance the body's ability to heal itself. Only through a comprehensive approach will the patient have the best chance of reversing his or her cancer.

"You can suppress the truth for only so long but eventually it will prove the perpetrators wrong." Dr. Gerald H. Smith

CHAPTER 8

INTEGRATIVE MEDICINES ROLE IN CANCER TREATMENT

Conventional Medicine vs Integrative Medicine

Conventional medicine's concept of integrative medicine is referring the patient to many different specialists in an attempt to solve the patient's problem. And when all else fails they send the patient to the psychiatrist because it must all be in their head. In contrast, true integrative medicine involves defining the underlying cause(s) of the "disease" process and integrating various modalities like light therapy, ozone, vitamins, minerals, homeopathics, osteopathic/chiropractic, Qigong acupuncture, and meditation, etc. to address the core issues. The approach is not just throwing darts at the patient or referring them to other specialists to just treat symptoms; conventional medicine's down fall will be the result of the consumer finally realizing their charade. In reality, conventional medicine doesn't know how to diagnose the underlying core problem; all they do is focus treatment on symptoms.

There is a saying, that the closer one gets to the truth the more simplistic the solution. After practicing over fifty years, this statement becomes more valid every day. The short coming of conventional medicine is that their curriculum does not teach this concept and has compartmentalized medicine into a group of super specialties. Pretty soon one will have to see a right kidney specialist vs a left kidney expert. The downside to integrative medicine is the fact that the educational curriculum does not encompass a broad scope of specialties. Integrative practitioners have to take many post-graduate seminars to gain the information. In my own case, it literally took me thirty-five years to piece the puzzle together. The other major problem is the fact that there are very few practitioners who know how it all fits together. At some point in the future, an organization like the World Organization For Natural Medicine will offer a comprehensive program to provide training in these numerous specialties. It requires a special person to make a dedicated commitment to learn this information.

The advantage of an integrative approach is that it views the patient globally and not just a bunch of symptoms. It was Sir William Osler who stated, "if you listen to the patient long enough, they will tell you the diagnosis." The first principle is to take a thorough medical history. Without a good patient background the practitioner has little if any guidance on what to evaluate. It's like someone wanting to drive to Los Angles from New York and they just drive West hoping they get close. The other major problem is the accuracy of the blood tests. A study on 2300 autopsy reports noted that the medical history accounted for 76% accuracy in making a correct diagnosis. In 12% of the patients, it was the physical findings that provided a correct diagnosis and disturbing was that only 11% of the patient's correct diagnosis was the direct result of the laboratory tests. Another disturbing fact was revealed when researchers from Mount Sinai Hospital compared basic blood tests from sixty healthy adults that were conducted at LabCorp, Quest Diagnostics, and Theranos; there were several cases where inaccurate results would have led to incorrect medical decisions. Medicine has to get back to basics. The old time family physician spent time examining his patient whereas today if your doctor spends three minutes with you you think you were blessed by the Pope.

Physicians have to check the patient's basic terrain by assessing their oral pH. A perfect example was a recent patient who came in with the chief complaints of joint pains especially in her hands and feet and vertigo. She was seen by numerous conventional doctors with no definitive diagnosis. An oral pH reading revealed a pH of 4.5 which is extremely acidic. A low pH lowers one's oxygen level, can easily cause vertigo, and damage one's DNA. Also an acidic terrain will lower one's pain threshold and metabolic wastes will cause joint pains. All the extensive blood testing just serves to drive up the patient's medical costs.

Of extreme importance is that cancer patients invariably are too acidic. Dr. Otto Warburg's Nobel Prize in Physiology defined the underlying cause for all cancers by showing an acid terrain causes anoxia. When my wife was in the hospital with stage III ovarian cancer, I asked her oncologist if he checks patient's pH. His response was it was not important. I then proceeded to tell him of Otto Warburg's Nobel Prize but he just blew it off. Another major pitfall of conventional medical doctors is their arrogance and their egos. The mind must be like a parachute. Both must be open in order to work.

Inquiring about exposures to chemicals is another crucial piece of information with cancer patients. One of my patients who had cancer in his lower left jawbone gave a history of chewing tobacco for 20 years and exposure to chemicals in the workplace. He also was undergoing dialysis for kidney failure. Quantum Testing revealed *Aspergillus terreus*, aluminum, and a pesticide, Terbufos. Unfortunately, the patient's toxicity burden was too great a factor and prevented his recovery.

Evaluating the teeth and jawbones is another often missed arena in cancer patients undergoing conventional treatment. A referred patient who had right lung cancer that metastasized to the left lung even after the cancer was surgically removed had an infected root canal tooth on the same side as the metastatic cancer. Once the "splinters," mercury, a pesticide, and cytomegalovirus were removed the cancer disappeared after six months of detox and removal of the infected tooth.

One of my patients who was diagnosed with acute myoloid leukemia gave a history of chemical exposure as a child; he stated that when he walked home from school he could taste the chemicals that were spewed out from a major chemical factory in his neighborhood. The chemicals became imbedded in his bone marrow and manifested later as an adult when his toxicity from teeth infections, chemtrail exposure, Lyme, trapped tetanus in his thyroid, presence of hypothyroidism, hypoadrenia, low testosterone level, and a pesticide carbryl overloaded his immune system. When I first examined the patient in May of 2014, he was given three months to live. Of interest, patients over 65 years of age with acute myoloid leukemia survive on average 2.4 months following chemotherapy. Ed survived five years following my recommended treatment plus other alternative approaches. What killed Ed in the end was the chemotherapy treatment he took. Poisoning the body never made any sense to me but because it generates over 450 billion dollars in revenue it provides a steady stream of income for many oncologists.

Liver Cancer

R.S. was a 72-year-old female patient diagnosed with hepatocellular carcinoma. The physician's report stated that the patient's lesion represented a metastatic disease that could be related to the carcinoma of the colon that was previously resected. The pathology report documented the presence of the cancer from the biopsy.

The patient refused conventional treatment of chemotherapy, radiation and surgery. The patient was placed on a nutritional regime that included a special herbal detox formula, glutathione, bromelain, and Livaplex. The patient's diet was modified to remove all fats, dairy products, and red meats. She was instructed to consume raw foods whenever possible (vegetables and seasonable fruits).

Three weeks after the nutritional therapy was initiated, the patient's constant liver pain completely resolved.

Laboratory Report:

Alkaline Phosphatase was 316 before vitamin therapy

Normal 40 to 150

Alkaline Phosphatase reduced to 193 three weeks following vitamin therapy

G-Glutamyl Transpeptadase was 359 before vitamin therapy

Normal 0 to 45

G-Glutamyl Transpeptadase reduced to 135 three weeks following vitamin therapy and further reduced to 69 four months post vitamin treatment

Remember that Cancer is Not a Disease. Cancer is an adaptation and survival mechanism that the body employs to stay alive. When the body is deprived of oxygen, the innate intelligence of the cell modifies its software allowing it to convert glucose into energy via a fermentation process (like in the production of wine or beer). Focusing and correcting the body's basic physiology allows the cells to return to normal.

Poor Quality of Life from Conventional Cancer Treatment

Joann was referred to my office by her doctor friend. Following the surgical removal of her cancerous thyroid Joann was placed on 125 mg of Synthroid (fourth most prescribed medication in the United States). This medication is a synthetic form of thyroxin and is not bio-equivalent to the natural hormone. Not a single cell in the human body can be "tricked" into considering them to be bio-equivalent. In some cases, Synthroid may actually worsen your condition. Synthroid only replaces T4, leaving your body to convert this to T3 (triiodothyronine, the biologically active form of the hormone). Most people cannot effectively convert the T4 in synthetic thyroid preparations to T3, which may explain why research has shown that a combination of T4 and T3 is often more effective than T4 alone. Synthroid is also a drug that is notoriously hard to prescribe and keep within the optimal dosage range.

Even though the patient was taking the Synthroid, she was still plagued with depression, anxiety, panic attacks, fatigue, dry hair, and brittle nails. Examination revealed the patient had toxicity issues with heavy metals, pesticides, and a virus. Placing Joann on a nutrient regime to detox her liver, open up her avenues of excretion, chelate out the heavy metals and pesticides and combat the infections. Within a week of starting her supplements, Joann witnessed a dramatic change. Her depression, anxiety and panic attacks disappeared, her energy increased as well as her sense of well-being. Zeroing in on the causative factors and removing them with natural food based nutrients allows the body to function more normally. Unfortunately for the patient, she most likely could have retained her thyroid gland if evaluated and treated with an integrated approach. Most often oncologists do not discuss with patients the poor quality of life that accompanies chemotherapy and the aspects of post-cancer chemotherapy treatment or the damage it inflicks. I guess their attitude is you are alive and you should be thankful.

Post-Cancer Treatment's Loss of Quality of Life

The one issue oncologists do not discuss with you is the loss of quality of life following chemotherapy. Their idea of successful treatment is killing the cancer. Unfortunately, the poison that they use has serious side effects which will rob you of energy, mental acuity, emotional stability, memory loss, and loss of that sense of well-being.

This was the case with Hallal. He had chemotherapy in 2010 for cancer and experienced post-treatment issues of chronic fatigue, emotional issues which included irritability and changes in mood. He also presented with several other medical complaints: chronic sciatic pain in his left hip and pain in his upper neck. There were two common denominators to all these issues: cranial distortions, which affected his entire spine and an underactive thyroid, which weakens muscles and ligaments and affected the function of his brain. An overlaying factor was the presence of pronated feet. Foot pronation invariably causes an ascending lesion up the spine causing upper cervical neck instability. A practitioner can treat the symptoms forever but until they define the underlying cause (pronated feet) the patient will never get rid of the pain and other symptoms.

When patients have a past history of chemotherapy, practitioners must focus on detoxing the body. Why? Because the toxic chemicals become trapped within the various tissues and organs of the body and cause dysfunction. One of the principal organs affected is the thyroid. Dysfunction of this organ was the source for this patient's mental and emotional state, muscle and ligament instability, lack of mental acuity, fatigue, and loss of that sense of well-being. An effective detox program resulted in dramatic changes for Hallal. His energy, mood swings, and sense of well-being improved tremendously. Adjustment of his cranium released tension down his spine and relieved his sciatic pain. Insertion of foot supports stabilized his pronation and helped alleviate his neck pain. The key to successful treatment is define the "splinters" and remove them. Unfortunately, conventional medicine has no understanding of how the body really works and their solution is to use drugs to the mask the symptoms.

PET Scan Documents Stage III Melanoma Reversal

Eliot flew up from Florida despite the admonitions of his daughter-in-law, who is a highly trained pediatric nurse, and his son. Getting a diagnosis of stage three melanoma in conventional medicine is like getting a death sentence.

After diagnosing the underlying "splinters," Eliot was placed on specific food-based supplements to detox his liver and address the causative factors. In addition, he was advised to purchase a home ozone unit and treat himself for 20 minutes a day. Of importance, Eliot was taking krill oil on a daily basis. Unfortunately, most people and physicians are not aware that **ALL fish** oils are rancid at room temperature. Ingesting rancid oils on a daily basis corrupts the cell membranes, lowers the oxygen intake and decreases energy production in the mitochondria within the cells. The result is congestive heart failure and cancer.

The following letter says it all.

Dear Dr Smith:

Surely God blessed me when I decided to place myself under your care. Let me explain. After foolishly neglecting a dark red blister on my thigh because it produced no discomfort, I finally decided to seek a professional opinion as the sore was not healing. A biopsy determined that I was in stage three melanoma. What a shocker! I was advised to seek help at the Sylvester Cancer Center in Miami, a renowned institution in this field. I was prescribed two drugs which were purported to halt the further progression of the disease. I was also advised that at least one third of the recipients of this medication receive major adverse side effects. Sadly, I was one of the "third." The reaction was so severe that I had to be rushed to the emergency room where I became very close to checking out.

Long story short, my options were few due to other existing conditions such as advanced age, COPD, hemolytic anemia and congestive heart failure to name a few. After recovering from the effects of the cancer meds, I did nothing hoping that the melanoma would just go away. Instead it progressed to a lymph node in the groin area resulting in major swelling and large purple pimples in the area. When I consulted the surgeon who removed the lesion on my leg, he said "You better get this attended to or you are going to die" Pretty scary huh?

That's when I made the game changing decision to see Dr. Smith. What's to lose? He proceeded to perform a series of tests the likes of which I never experienced. He then placed me on a regimen of dietary supplements which nobody ever heard of with some ozone therapy thrown in for good measure. Well here I am, a couple of months later, ecstatic to report that so far the swelling in the groin has all but disappeared and the ugly purple pimples are almost all faded away, that is not to mention feeling better in general.

Before I ramble on endlessly, let me close by saying that as time goes on, more and more of us will realize that natural healing is the way to go. God bless you Dr. Gerry and the good work that you do."

Basis for All Cancers: Adulterated Omega 6 oils

In essence, cancer is **NOT** a disease. It is a breakdown of the immune system and corruption of the cell membranes by adulterated omega 6 oils which prevent adequate levels of oxygen to pass into the cell. It is the organic, cold press omega-6 component that acts as a magnet pulling in the oxygen into the cell. When the oxygen level drops by 35%, the cell goes into survival mode. Low oxygen initiates fermentation which converts glucose into lactic acid. Over time the cells transform into cancer cells. The solution is simple: supply organic, cold pressed omega-6 fatty acid to rebuild the cell membrane and detox the other toxins (heavy metals, chemicals, vaccines and their adjuvants, viruses and the pathogens, herbicides, etc.) which further corrupt the cell membrane.

Stage IV Lung Cancer markedly improved in two months

Most people lose it when they get a diagnosis of the Big "C". Not Deborah a 64-year-old feisty Canadian resident. She viewed her diagnosis as a life changing event and became extremely proactive. The following is a brief overview of her commitment to get well:

- Twice weekly intravenous Vitamin C at 75 g per treatment
- Avemar from Hungary (Fermented Wheat Germ Extract)
- Predominantly plant based diet
- Far Infra-Red Sauna Detox
- Attempt to alkalize body
- Meditation
- Removed some stressors from life personal and work

- Pancreatic enzymes
- Supplements - turmeric, selenium, magnesium, D3, K2, K3, Quercetin, Mushrooms, ALA

My e-mail response to Deborah's initial inquiry was, "What you are doing is admirable and shows your commitment to getting well however you are just throwing darts and hoping they will hit the cancer." My approach is much more precise. Define the potential stressors: dental (root canal teeth, mercury fillings, cavitation in post-extraction wisdom teeth or other sites, galvanic currents, toxic dental materials, cranial stress patterns, dental malocclusion causing an autonomic imbalance), in the thyroid (vaccines, pesticides, heavy metals, liver, brain, etc.), then define specific natural food based supplements to remove the stressors.

In my 50 plus years practicing, I have found this to be the most effective means of treating disease. All other approaches are just guessing and all the sophisticated blood testing does not tell you what the underlying cause(s) are. Unfortunately, most physicians have been dumb down and patients are fed much disinformation and given a distorted view of cancer, which then creates fear so they will accept the conventional dogma of chemo, surgery, and radiation. All of the above is constantly being reinforced by the 11 O'clock news, all cancer societies, oncologists, and other governing bodies.

The following was a brief medical history:

- July 25-2016 diagnosed with stage II lung cancer.
- September 11, 2016 surgery to remove lower right lobe containing 3.3 cm tumor as well as two impacted lymph nodes within the lobe. **Declared cancer free. This is the big lie. Cutting out the cancer does NOT address the causative factors!**
- June 12, 2017 cancer returns in all lobes (0.2 to 0.3 cm tumors mainly + one 1.5 cm tumor). The surgery caused the stage II cancer to become a stage IV malignancy.
- June 16-2017 malignant pleurisy drainage required every 3 weeks but nearly cleared.
- Coughing, shortness of breath and pain in bones.

- July 11-2017 started GIOTRIF; (afatinib tablets) 3rd generation targeted therapy drug which has restored lifestyle by removing the cough, breath and pain but it only works for 6-18 months and has many unpleasant side effects.
- **The patient was totally misled when told she was cancer free.** Cutting out the symptom, tumor, is not addressing the underlying cause(s) of the disease process. It's like painting over rust. It just buys you a little time before the rust pops up somewhere else.

The patient was placed on Synthroid. My response was, "Synthroid often does not work leaving a weak immune system. With a weak immune system any disease will have a greater chance of returning. Must define what is in your thyroid preventing it from working and not prescribe a hormone which will not solve the underling problem plus Synthroid will shut down the thyroid. Also every supplement must be tested for energetic compatibility. One can be taking the best supplements in the world but if the energy pattern of the supplements does not match that of the patient the results are often disappointing."

My initial evaluation on August 29, 2017 revealed that Deborah's thyroid had, mercury, lead, cadmium, aluminum, arsenic, cytomegalovirus, Epstein Barr virus, a vaccine, and several pesticides. A nutritional protocol including special sequencing of supplements was established to remove the offending items. In addition, Deborah was treated with cranial manipulation, scalar energy and soft laser.

Deborah returned two months later on October 24, 2017 for a follow-up visit. She showed me her scan results which stated a 47% reduction in tumor size (1.7cm reduced to .9mm) in just two months. Plus the cancer in her pleural lining surrounding the lungs was almost totally resolved. Deborah's energy is through the roof and her activities have not been curtailed.

As with all disease processes, the underlying causative factors must be uncovered. Then appropriate therapies must be custom designed to meet the specific needs of the patient. Deborah's testimonial demonstrates the efficacy of a comprehensive approach. Available at https://www.icnr.com/cs/cs_100.html.

"It is better to walk alone, than with a crowd going in the wrong direction"

Herman Siu

CHAPTER 9

RECONSTRUCTING MITOCHONDRIA, DNA, AND HEALING

Discovery of Biophotons

In 1923, the Russian and Soviet scientist Alexander Gurwitsch discovered a morphogenetic field governing biological development, he called the phenomenon mitogenetic radiation. This concept provided the basis for Dr. Fritz Albert Popp's discovery of biophotons in the 1970s, and provided the basis for Dr. Bruce Lipton's concepts of his Biology of Belief. As Dr. Lipton states, it is the environmental influences that dictate the cells reaction. In essence, it is the morphogenetic field that acts as the sensor for environmental stimuli.

Dr. Popp discovered that carcinogens "scrambled" light with a wavelength of 380 nanometers whereas benign chemicals do not. When cells are exposed to very weak UV light, particularly that with a wavelength of 380 nanometers they quickly self-repair. Popp hypothesized that cancer results from a disruption of the cells' photorepair system. Interestingly, the presence of carcinogens, which block the healing wavelength of 380 nm, adulterated oils, which corrupt the cell membranes reducing absorption of oxygen, a +55 millivolt cell membrane potential that triggers cell proliferation, a processed food diet which is low in biophotons and nutrients, plus a mix of pathogens, vaccines and chemical toxins all combine to form the perfect storm - cancer.

The key to restoring cellular health is to raise the level of biophotons, which Popp and his student Bernard Ruth found in all living systems: mitochondria, DNA, cells, and tissues through out our body. This stored light is released as very weak, extremely coherent biophotons, which trigger off the 100,000 chemical reactions a second in each cell. When a biophoton is taken up into the chemical reaction it does so with very little release of heat. At the completion of the reaction, the biophoton is released back into the morphogenic field and waits to catalyze the next reaction. One biophoton is capable of trigger off 100,000 chemical reactions.

The electromagnetic field surrounding the cell produces a spatial dynamic pattern, which in turn acts as the dispatcher providing the information to tell the cells what to do, at what time, and at what place. Biophotons have a very high degree of coherence; the higher the degree of coherence the more stable the electromagnetic pattern and the more it is predictable. This is the characteristic and signature of coherence.

In his many years of research, Popp found that biophoton emissions from healthy humans display rhythmic patterns. He also observed that the coherence of the emissions, the intensity, and the rhythmic patterns varied in people with different illnesses. For example, people with multiple sclerosis, absorb too much light and their photon emissions display too much order. Biophoton emissions from cancer patients lack coherence and fail to follow natural rhythmic patterns. Also, tumors emit high amounts of photons: an average of 300 or 90 photons/cm per minute compared with normal tissue that emits an average of 22 or 6 photons/cm per minute. Popp and colleagues at the International Institute of Biophysics have discovered that surface tumors and tumors excised during surgery respond to remedies which change the photon emissions of the cancer. Most chemical/drug treatments have no effect on the tumor's high emission rate. However, when a nontoxic remedy with decreased emissions is applied, the tumor responds to that agent and will most likely improve the patient's condition and may even promote a cure. Rather than killing tumor cells, the beneficial agent appears to stimulate the abnormal cell to revert back to its factory default settings and function as a healthy cell.

Levels of Oxidative Stress Alters the Level of Biophotons

Free radicals, as that produced from the conversion of food to energy, are missing one electron; in order to become stable, they must steal an electron from a stable source like your DNA, lipids, or proteins. The presence of free radicals stimulates more biophotons. Exposure to the sun stresses your skin, which in turn causes the release of more biophotons to deal with the reactions.

Communication

Dr. Bruce Lipton is correct when he says the cells react to our environment. In contrast, taking antioxidant supplements like quercetin or CoQ_{10} reduce the quantity of biophotons. These biophotons are the messengers that make up the communications network among cells. It is easy to understand that if this communication system gets disrupted then the cell physiology becomes dysfunctional. This is one reason to include fresh raw foods and food based supplements into your diet; they supply biophotons to insure healthy cells. Synthetic vitamins and processed foods supply no biophotons.

Interesting is the research into biophotons' role in communication inside and outside your body. At base, what is now known is that your cells' DNA not only emits light, but it absorbs it, as well. The experimental implication is that biophotons are a means of communication among your cells, communication that occurs at the speed of light — 186,000 miles per second. It is now generally accepted that the coordination among cells in your body, coordination that happens within milliseconds and even shorter times, is orchestrated by biophotons.

Integrative medicine utilizes many different modalities to heal the body. One such technology involves use of biophotons (packets of light energy emitted by the sun and stored in raw food and DNA) from the UV light spectrum.

Dr. Fritz Albert Popp, a German theoretical biophysicist credited with the discovery of biophotons, showed that when cancer cells were illuminated with a method called photo repair, a weaker intensity of UV light caused the DNA to undergo rapid healing. It is only when UV light is at a lower intensity level that the healing of DNA occurs.

Dr. Popp built a machine called the "photomultiplier" which measures weak photon emissions that stimulate healing. While measuring these photons in humans, he discovered that the cells of the body have biological rhythms of 7, 14, 32, 80, and 270 days respectively. It also showed that people who had these disturbed biological rhythms were cancer patients. His research also showed that stress triggered an increase in biophotons, which in the short term was beneficial to good health.

It is no surprise that foods highest in biophotons are also used as natural cancer cures, especially when you eat them within 3 hours after being picked from the ground. Dr. Gabriel Cousens states that people who have a junk food diet register 1,000 or less biophotons in their system, whereas people eating a fresh raw food diet have 83,000 or more biophotons in their body.

Mechanism Why Carinogens Cause Cancer

In the 1970s, Dr. Popp discovered that all carcinogens, like formaldehyde or fluoride, prevent the body from absorbing the wavelenghth of 380 nm to repair the DNA. This process triggers degeneration and disease. This blocking effect holds true for all carcinogens and prevents the DNA from repairing. Popp's concept states, "the function of our entire metabolism is dependent on light." These weaken emitted light, from our body is in fact responsible for our mental, physical and emotional health. The effect of wi-fi, EMFs, and especially 5G radiation directly disturbs our aura or more correctly our morphogenic field, which in turn causes the cells to respond to such stimuli. A perfect illustration is seen in the direct effect of this author's discovery of the TESLA ENERGY CARD™. The magnetic strip can be imprinted with specific healing frequencies. When the card is placed in contact with the body, its frequencies penetrate into the tissues and organs. The two infrared photographs depict a positive change in the body within five minutes. The pre-treatment photograph represents a baseline depicting a blue or cold temperature over the area of the left lobe of the patient's thyroid with a temperature reading of 35.20 C. The second infrared photograph documents a shift to a warmer, more yellow color temperature which was recorded at 35.30 C. The initial experiment was conducted to test the influence of the healing frequencies of the TESLA ENERGY CARD® against the presence of two pathogens, cytomegalovirus and

Epstein Barr virus, originally diagnosed in the lobe of the patient's left thyroid. Immediately following the five-minute treatment session, the patient stated that, "she felt calmer." Also of interest was that using the Quantum Testing Technique, the area tested negative when both test vials of the two pathogens were placed directly over the area where the two viruses previously tested positive. This result signifies that the frequency field of the viruses were altered to negate their toxic frequency.

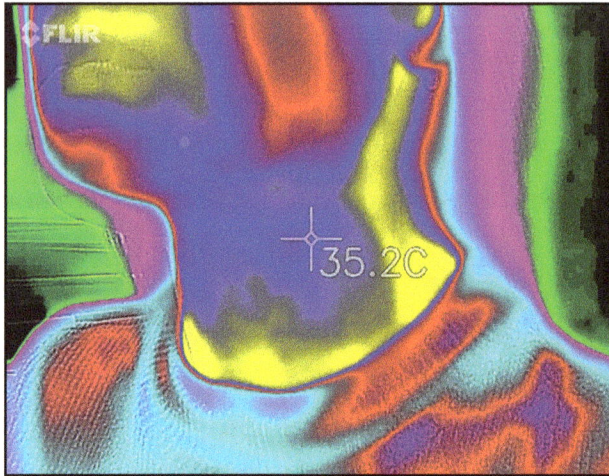

Pre-Treatment	Post-Treatment

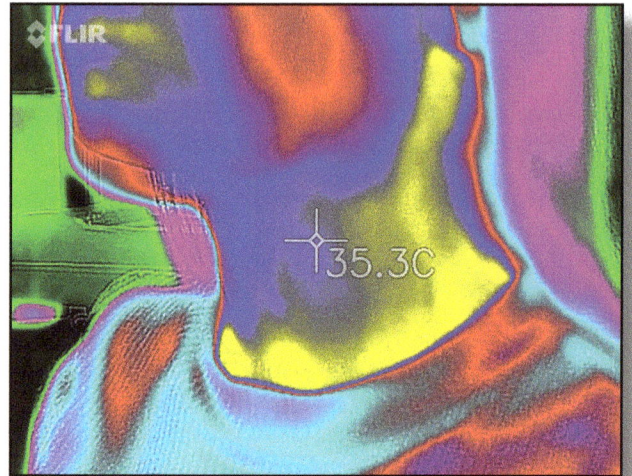

Dr. Fritz Alber Popp stated that in each cell of our body 100,000 chemical reactions are occurring every second. These chemical reactions are initiated by biophotons. Cells only need one biophoton to trigger off 100,000 chemical reactions. Many of these chemical reactions are taking place in the mitochondria within each cell.

The mitochondria are unique intracellular structures that produce 95% of the cellular energy and plays a critical role in protecting the cell from oxidative stress. They are the powerhouse of the cell and are the only intracellular organelle that has its own DNA and is able to divide and replicate on its own. Most cells have anywhere from 1 to 2,000 of them. In heart muscle cells, about 40% of the cytoplasmic space is taken up by mitochondria. In liver cells, the figure is about 20-25% with 1000 to 2000 mitochondria per cell. A large amount of adenosine triphosphate (ATP) must be produced by the mitochondria every second of every day because ATP cannot be stored. This function is so important that mitochondria can take up as much as 25% of the cell volume.

Importance of mitochondrial dysfunction

The general consensus among researchers is that mitochondrial dysfunction plays a central role in nearly every degenerative disease and especially in cancer. The major factors involved in poor mitochondrial function include deficiencies in critical cellular nutrients, proprioceptive deficiencies, and environmental toxicity. The standard American diet, sedentary lifestyle, and ubiquitous amount of toxins in our society make today's generation far more susceptible for mitochondrial dysfunction than ever before. Mitochondrial dysfunction is directly related to excess fatigue especially among cancer patients. In addition to the above factors, many commonly used drugs damage the mitochondria: acetaminophen (Tylenol), antibiotics, aspirin, AZT, cocaine, indomethacin, L-DOPA, NSAIDs, and statin drugs (Lipitor and Crestor). Reduced energy ultimately translates into an acid terrain which lowers oxygen levels, damages DNA and initiates cancer. Many of the adverse events associated with these prescriptions are well explained by the mitochondrial dysfunction they induce, secondary to depletion of a major antioxidant nutrient, CoQ10. It is not surprising that statins increase all-cause mortality and most chronic disease. The research on alcohol is clear. The more you consume, the greater the depletion of NADH* needed for Adenosine triphosphate (ATP) production. Without energy the immune system begins to shut down.

* Nicotinamide adenine dinucleotide dehydrogenase is an enzyme that is a part of the mitochondrial respiratory chain, which catalyzes transfer of electrons from NADH to ubiquinone (CoQ_{10}).

Dietary Supplements Commonly Used for Primary Mitochondrial Disease

The most commonly used dietary supplement ingredients for Primary Mitochondrial Disorders include antioxidants, such as vitamin C, vitamin E, and alpha-lipoic acid; electron donors and acceptors, such as CoQ10 and riboflavin; compounds that can be used as alternative energy sources, such as creatine; and compounds that can conjugate or bind mitochondrial toxins, such as carnitine, glutathione, methionine, and methyl sulfonyl methane (MSM).

The foundation begins with a good food based multivitamin and mineral. They should be of high quality with 2 to 3 times the recommended daily intake for most nutrients, especially the B vitamins. Of all the mitochondrial supportive nutrients, at the top of my list are (in order of my preference) CoQ10, α-lipoic acid plus acetyl-l-carnitine, resveratrol, NAC, and vitamin E. Also of value are extra virgin coconut oil, pyrroloquinoline quinone (PQQ), Ginkgo biloba, proanthocyanidins, and melatonin.

CoQ10

This supplement is an antioxidant present in all cells and particularly concentrated in the mitochondria. CoQ10 participates in the production of adenosine triphosphate (ATP)—the high-energy packets that fuel our minds and bodies—as part of the electron transport chain and also protects the mitochondria against free-radical damage.

α-Lipoic Acid + Acetyl-l-Carnitine

These nutrients have been used together to increase mitochondrial ATP production in several animal models, including elderly animals in particular. Human research is starting to show the same benefits. (200 mg of α-lipoic acid and 500 mg of acetyl-l-carnitine 2X/day). **Alpha lipoic acid** also called lipoic acid or ALA is also important for promoting mitochondrial biogenesis. ALA also helps with blood sugar and weight control because it stimulates glucose uptake and increases the burning of fatty acids. I recommend 600–1,200 mg of ALA daily.

Resveratrol

Resveratrol increases mitochondrial ATP production, protects from reactive oxygen species (ROS), up-regulates sirtuin*, and so forth. It even clears β-amyloid plaque from Alzheimer's disease cells. Human studies are now confirming animal studies showing improved mitochondrial functional at surprisingly reasonable dosages. (150 mg 4X/day.)

N-Acetyl Cysteine (NAC)

The key role of NAC is to increase intracellular glutathione, which is then pumped into the mitochondria. This glutathione is critical for protection of mitochondria from oxidative damage. (500 mg 2X/day.)

* Sirtuins are a family of proteins that regulate cellular health. Sirtuins play a key role in regulating cellular homeostasis. Homeostasis involves keeping the cell in balance. However, sirtuins can only function in the presence of NAD+, nicotinamide adenine dinucleotide, a coenzyme found in all living cells.

Vitamin E

Extensive cell and animal research showing that the antioxidant vitamin E protects mitochondria from oxidative stress. The human research is not as strong and unfortunately is almost all with a single member of the vitamin E family. Nonetheless, there are promising early results. (Mixed tocopherols 500 IU 1X/day.)

Zinc Orotate

The orotate form is easily absorbed into the tissues. When zinc enters the cell it prevents the replication of viruses thus boosting the immune system. It's also essential in DNA and protein synthesis and in enzyme reactions. Zinc is naturally found in a wide variety of both plant and animal foods.

Magnesium Orotate

Plays an important role in a wide variety of biochemical processes including optimizing mitochondrial function. The evidence is clear: if you want to optimize your mitochondrial function, metabolism, and reduce your risk for type 2 diabetes and cardiovascular disease, one of the things you need to do is consume adequate magnesium. Magnesium also plays a role in your body's detoxification processes and therefore is important for helping to prevent damage from environmental chemicals, heavy metals, and other toxins.

Vitamin D

Great mitochondrial boosting nutrient by maintaining mitochondrial integrity and cell metabolism. Regulates calcium homeostasis. Good for xenobiotic (a chemical compound foreign to a given biological system) detoxification. Protects cells from excessive respiration and production of reactive oxygen species that leads to cell damage. Vitamin D is essential for the health of all human tissues.

Folic Acid

Folic Acid functions in enzyme complexes participating in mitochondrial respiration and energy production or they are required for synthesis of mitochondrial respiratory chain components. There is evidence supporting the association between low folate status and mitochondrial DNA (mtDNA) instability, and cerebral folate deficiency is relatively frequent in mitochondrial disorders.

Clinician's Preference (11:1 ratio of omega 6 to omega 3 organic, cold pressed oils)

Adulterated omega 6 oil in the diet corrupts the cell membranes transforming them into plastic. They are also pro-inflammatory. A corrupted cell membrane prevents waste products from exiting and nutrients and oxygen from entering the cell. This is a major missing link in the degenerative disease equation and especially important in cancer cells.

Glutathione

The body's most powerful antioxidant that has even been called "the master antioxidant," requires magnesium for its synthesis. This antioxidant is essential in the detox process, chelates heavy metals and toxins, supports the immune system, helps regenerate vitamin C and E, helps make DNA, and is anti-inflammatory.

Zymessence

This is a systemic enzyme versus a digestive enzyme. It is anti-inflammatory, reduces fibrosis or scarring, which results from chronic inflammation. It is anti-bacterial, mildly antiviral, it digests foreign protein in the blood and can digest the biofilm secreted by cancer cells.

L-Arginine

It is an amino acid that is the primary precursor of nitric oxide (NO)—one of several biochemical pathways that are powered up by exercise. In addition to its protective effects on the mitochondria, NO is a very powerful vasodilator. It relaxes the arteries, enhances vascular health, improves blood flow, and even boosts sexual function. The suggested dose of L-arginine is 1,000–2,000 mg a day.

Based on my 50 plus years of clinical experience I strongly recommend that each supplement be tested for biocompatibility with the patient and dosage. I am not a proponent of using standard protocols. In other words, one size does not fit all.

When the conventional medical establishment feels threatened by non-drug therapies and they realize they are losing market share, they start publishing articles in professional journals and/or lay magazines targeting energy/integrated medicine and even go so far as describing it as "Quackery." The Encyclopedia Britannica defines quackery "as the characteristic practice of quacks or charlatans, who pretend to knowledge and skill that they do not possess, particularly in medicine." The following information is presented for your perusal to help you better define medical quackery.

- Since 1971, when President Nixon declared a "War on Cancer" over 500 billion dollars have been spent on cancer research. To date the cancer rates have gotten worse not better.

- A review of the gold standard of medical literature reveals that the five-year cancer survival rate for chemotherapy in the US is 2.1% and 2.3% success in Australia. This is after 51 years of research and over 500 billion dollars invested.

- The estimated total number of iatrogenic deaths–that is, deaths induced inadvertently by a physician or surgeon or by medical treatment or diagnostic procedures– in the US annually is 783,936. It is evident that the American medical system is itself the leading cause of death and injury in the US.

- Simply entering a hospital could result in the following:
  - In 16.4 million people, a 2.1% chance (affecting 186,000) of a serious adverse drug reaction
  - In 16.4 million people, a 5–6% chance (affecting 489,500) of acquiring a health-care acquired infection
  - In 16.4 million people, a 4–36% chance (affecting 1.78 million) of having an iatrogenic injury (medical error and adverse drug reactions).
  - In 16.4 million people, a 17% chance (affecting 1.3 million) of a procedure error.

These statistics were compiled and verified and published in an article:

Death by Medicine
By Gary Null, PhD; Carolyn Dean MD, ND; Martin Feldman, MD;
Debora Rasio, MD; and Dorothy Smith, PhD
Published in Life Extension magazine March 2004

- Richard Horton, ex-editor of the internationally prestigious medical journal Lancet stated, "bluntly that major pharmaceutical companies falsify or manipulate tests on the health, safety, and effectiveness of their various drugs by taking samples too small to be statistically meaningful or hiring test labs or scientists where the lab or scientist has blatant conflicts of interest such as pleasing the drug company to get further grants."

Quackery "is the characteristic practice of quacks or charlatans, who pretend to knowledge and skill that they do not possess, particularly in medicine."

"All truth passes through three stages. First, it is ridiculed. Second, it is violently opposed. Third, it is accepted as being self-evident." *Arthur Schopenhauer* (1788-1860)

"Most of the things worth doing in the world had been declared **IMPOSSIBLE** before they were done." Louis D. Brandeis

Conventional medicine is under attack because its paradigm is obsolete, its research is fraudulent, its drugs are too expensive and kill at least 106,000 people a year from adverse reactions from properly prescribed FDA approved drugs, and they are losing market share because people are slowly waking up to the ruse.

"The art of medicine consists in amusing the patient while nature cures the disease."
Voltaire

CHAPTER 10

NUTRITIONAL SURVIVAL GUIDE FOR CANCER

The average person welcomes a basic primer on nutrition to guide them through the maze of the best foods to consume and the ones to void. The basic objective is to establish a healthy terrain in which pathogens (viruses, bacteria, mold, and fungi), and cancer cannot survive. People do NOT get sick because of viruses like COVID-19 or get attacked by cancer; they get sick and get cancer because their body's terrain becomes toxic, which allows the bugs to flourish and cancer to initiate.

Health involves a lifestyle change. Grocery shelves are packed with foods containing high fructose corn syrup, food additives, preservatives, MSG, colored dyes, sodium benzoate, and many more poisons. Consuming these foods will increase your insulin levels, which in turn causes wide spread inflammation and fibrosis (scarring) solidifying your organs, clogging your arteries, decreasing circulation in your brain (dementia), and create many symptoms and premature death. To guide people in their detox journey, I have formulated a sequence of six phases of detoxification that will establish a healthy terrain.

Detox

After 35 years of clinical observation and research, the following sequence for detoxification was formulated to streamline the process and help reduce herxheimer's reactions:

Phase I: Detox the liver, kidneys, intestines, lungs, and other tissues.

Phase II: Open up the avenues of excretion by means of homeopathic remedies.

Phase III: Remove any heavy metals.

Phase IV: Remove herbicides, pesticides, and insecticides.

Phase V: Resolve infections.

Phase VI: Detox any vaccines.

It must also be emphasized that during the detox process one must consume real foods (organic vegetables like kale, collard greens, carrots, cilantro, celery, seaweeds; grass-fed meats, raw milk, raw juices, and raw nuts and sprouted seeds). The body in its infinite wisdom has the capacity to heal itself if it is given the raw materials. Pop tarts and other devitalized foods do not supply the raw nutrients to heal. In fact, these devitalized foods present a burden to the body because much energy and nutrients are wasted to remove these poisons.

The philosophy is simple. Since the blood of the entire body filters through the liver every three minutes, it is imperative to cleanse the main filter first and give it the proper nutrients it needs to process the toxins it pulls out of the blood. If the liver cannot process the toxins they will keep recirculating until they get trapped in other organs or tissues. Once the filter is cleaned out, the the avenues of excretion must be opened up. A free flowing filter can now handle the increased dumping of toxins. Next, the heavy metals must be removed. Heavy metals impede cellular function and suppress the immune system. With a clean filter and drainage system working, it's time to remove the herbicides, insecticides, pesticides, and other chemicals. All the above help establish a stronger immune system. The body can now fight any infections more effectively. With all the potential major burdens reduced, the immune system can direct more of its energies to expel any trapped vaccines, drugs and other stored toxins. This approach is the most logical and dramatically reduces any incidences of herxheimer reaction. The end result is that the body has been reset to "factory default" and can function more normally.

Why Go Organic: The No. 1 reason people go organic is to avoid pesticides, chemicals and all of those things that are not allowed in organics. Eating nonorganic genetically modified foods (GMOs) is associated with higher glyphosate levels and reduced nutrients in your body. Even if you buy organic, glyphosate has been found in the rain water and literally contaminates everything.

There are three basic food groups: fats, protein, and carbohydrates. There are good and bad components within each group. Genetically modified foods like canola seeds (derived from modified rapeseeds) become toxic when processed into canola oil are toxic. They were genetically modified to withstand the treatment of herbicides like glyphosate, aka Round-Up, a Monsanto herbicide, which is known to cause cancer. Adulterated oils like canola, soy, cotton seed, corn, safflower, and sunflower literally change the fats in your cell membranes into plastic. This is one major reason why there are so many degenerative diseases (diabetes, cardiovascular, and cancer) today. A plastic membrane prevents the uptake of oxygen and nutrients into the cell and removal of wastes out of the cell. In addition, canola oil is a long chain fatty acid (18 or more carbons), which causes it to go rancid in your liver.

Protein

Interestingly, mother's milk is composed mainly of fats and proteins with no carbohydrates. One should focus on consuming good proteins and fats just as Mother Nature intended. Any animal protein should be grass fed, no antibiotics, no steroids, or growth hormones. The big advantage is that animal protein helps repair your body, boosts your immune system, and helps keep your blood sugar high for longer periods.

Why Eat Animal Protein?: Research published in the journal Nutrition shows that those who eat a strictly plant-based diet may suffer from subclinical protein malnutrition, which means they also are likely not getting enough dietary sulfur. Sulfur is the third most abundant mineral in the human body. It is derived almost exclusively from dietary protein, such as fish and high-quality (organic and/or grass-fed/pastured) beef and poultry. Meat and fish are considered "complete" as they contain all the sulfur-containing amino acids you need to produce new protein.

Needless to say, those who abstain from animal protein are placing themselves at far greater risk of sulfur deficiency and its related health problems. Sulfur also plays a vital role in the structure and biological activity of both proteins and enzymes. If you don't have sufficient amounts of sulfur in your body, this deficiency can cascade into a number of health problems as it will affect bones, joints, connective tissues, metabolic processes, and more.

1. Avoiding animal foods may lead to a low dietary intake of protein and sulfur amino acids, which puts anyone avoiding animal foods at an increased risk of cardiovascular diseases.
2. Those who abstain from animal protein are at far greater risk of sulfur deficiency which is vitally important for muscle strength and detoxification.
3. Animal foods from healthy, appropriately raised sources, such as organic, grass- fed meat, raw milk, and free-range eggs, are loaded with healthy nutrients like sulfur, which are highly beneficial for heart health.

Protein Payout: 4 oz strip steak, 133 calories, 26 g protein

When it comes to steak or burgers, go grass-fed. It may ding your wallet, but it'll dent your abs. Grass-fed beef is naturally leaner and has fewer calories than conventional meat: A lean seven-ounce conventional strip steak has 386 calories and 16 grams of fat. But a seven-ounce grass-fed strip steak has only 234 calories and five grams of fat. Grass-fed meat also contains higher levels of omega-3 fatty acids, according to a study published in the Nutrition Journal, which have been shown to reduce the risk of heart disease.

Sources of quality protein: Boneless and Skinless Chicken or Turkey Breast. You want to make sure they were not fed antibiotics, growth hormones, and steroids.

Fish. Avoid farm raised fish because they are fed genetically modified foods. Also certain fish are high in mercury: grouper, tuna, swordfish, shark, king mackerel, tilefish, marlin, orange roughy, striped bass, and mahi-mahi.

The following fish are low in mercury:

- Freshwater perch
- Sardines
- Salmon: wild caught

- Skate
- Canned light tuna (skipjack)
- American and spiny lobster
- Jacksmelt
- Boston or chub mackerel
- Trout
- Squid
- Whitefish
- American shad
- Crab
- Scallop
- Catfish
- Mullet
- Flounder, fluke, plaice, sand dabs
- Herring
- Anchovies
- Pollock
- Crawfish
- Hake

Legumes: lima beans, black beans, chickpeas, pinto beans, kidney beans, lentils, peas, navy beans.

Grains: barley, brown rice, buckwheat, bulgur (cracked wheat), millet, oatmeal, corn, kalmut, rye, semolina wheat, spelt, triticale, sorghum, farro, teff (is a food high in phosphorus; teff also serves as a natural remedy for PMS and cramps; and it's gluten-free), wheat, and fonio.

Important Notes: Eating whole grains is **NOT** as healthy as one might think. One of the major downsides of eating grains is that they contain anti-nutrients like gliadin, an immunotoxic protein. It is capable of increasing the production of another intestinal protein zonulin, which in turn opens up gaps in the normally tight junctures between intestinal cells. In lay terms this is called "leaky gut," which causes chronic inflammation.

Wheat Germ Agglutinin (WGA)

Another toxic component present in grains is lectins. Wheat germ agglutinin (WGA) is a particularly resilient and problematic lectin. It is not eliminated through sprouting and is actually found in higher concentrations in whole wheat. Studies indicate that it has the potential to contribute to a wide range of adverse health effects, including gut inflammation and damage to your gastrointestinal tract.

Pro-inflammatory—WGA stimulates the synthesis of pro-inflammatory chemical messengers (cytokines) in intestinal and immune cells, and has been shown to play a causative role in chronic gut inflammation.

Immunotoxicity—WGA causes the thymus gland to shrink in rats, and anti-WGA antibodies in human blood have been shown to cross-react with other proteins. This indicates that they may contribute to autoimmunity. In fact, WGA appears to play a role in celiac disease (CD) that is entirely distinct from that of gluten, revealed by significantly higher levels of IgG and IgA antibodies against WGA found in patients with CD, when compared with patients with other intestinal disorders.

Neurotoxicity—WGA can cross your blood-brain barrier through a process called "adsorptive endocytosis," pulling other substances with it. WGA may attach to your myelin sheath and is capable of inhibiting nerve growth factor, which is important for the growth, maintenance, and survival of certain target neurons.

Excitotoxicity—WGA present in wheat, dairy, and soy contain exceptionally high levels of glutamic and aspartic acid, which makes them all potentially excitotoxic. Excitotoxicity is a damaging process where glutamic and aspartic acid cause an over-activation of your nerve cell receptors. This can lead to calcium-induced nerve and brain injury. These two amino acids may contribute to neurodegenerative conditions such as multiple sclerosis, Alzheimer's, Huntington's disease, and other nervous system disorders such as epilepsy, ADD/ADHD and migraines.

Cytotoxicity—WGA has been demonstrated to be cytotoxic to both normal and cancerous cell lines, capable of inducing either cell cycle arrest or programmed cell death (apoptosis).

Disrupts Endocrine Function—WGA may contribute to weight gain, insulin resistance, and leptin resistance by blocking the leptin receptor in your hypothalamus. It also binds to both benign and malignant thyroid nodules, and interferes with the production of secretin from your pancreas, which can lead to digestive problems and pancreatic enlargement.

Cardiotoxicity—WGA has a potent, disruptive effect on platelet endothelial cell adhesion molecule-1 which plays a key role in tissue regeneration and safely removing neutrophils from your blood vessels.

WGA Adversely Affects Gastrointestinal Function by causing increased shedding of the intestinal brush border membrane, reducing the surface area, and accelerating cell loss and shortening of villi. It also causes degradation in intestinal cells, contributing to cell death and increased turnover, and decreases levels of heat shock proteins in gut epithelial cells, leaving them more vulnerable to damage.

As noted earlier, the highest amount of WGA is found in whole wheat, including its sprouted form, which is touted as being the most healthful form of all … The traditional ways of addressing many of these anti-nutrients is, in fact, by sprouting, fermenting and cooking. However, lectins are designed to withstand degradation through a wide range of pH and temperatures. WGA lectin is particularly tough because it's actually formed by the same disulfide bonds that give strength and resiliency to vulcanized rubber and human hair.

As you might suspect, leaky gut can cause digestive symptoms such as bloating, gas and abdominal cramps, but it can also cause or contribute to many others you may not be aware of, such as fatigue, skin rashes, joint pain, allergies, psychological symptoms, autism and more. It's a vicious cycle because once your digestive tract has been damaged, it allows various gut contents to flood into your bloodstream where they wreak havoc on your health. The key to preventing this lies in altering your diet to eliminate the offending foods — including sugars and grains — as well as introducing healthier ones that will support a proper balance of bacteria in your gut. To restore gut health and prevent leaky gut from occurring, it is essential to eat traditionally fermented foods.

Dr. Natasha Campbell-McBride explains: "Fermented foods are essential to introduce, as they provide probiotic microbes in the best possible form … fermented foods will carry probiotic microbes all the way down to the end of the digestive system. Fermentation predigests the food, making it easy for our digestive systems to handle, that is why fermented foods are easily digested by people with damaged gut. Fermentation releases nutrients from the food, making them more bio-available for the body: for example, sauerkraut contains 20 times more bio-available vitamin C than fresh cabbage."

On Dr. Campbell-McBride's web site (www.gaps.me/dr-campbell-mcbride.php) you can find recipes for many traditionally fermented foods, including sauerkraut, yogurt, kefir, kvass and more.

If you regularly eat fermented foods such as these that have not been pasteurized (pasteurization kills the naturally occurring probiotics), your healthy gut bacteria will thrive. If these foods do not make a regular appearance in your diet, or you've recently taken antibiotics, a high-quality probiotic supplement will help give your gut bacteria the healthy boost it needs. Once your gut flora is optimized, your leaky gut should improve naturally. As Dr. Cordain explains: *"… when we have a healthy flora of bacteria in our gut, it tends to prevent leaky gut."*

Why Raw Milk? Raw milk is fast becoming the number one hot food topic and has emerged as a high priority health food in America. People need and want clean raw milk that is produced in organic, grass-fed conditions. Raw milk retains its enzymes, good grass-fed fats, and wonderful, bio-diverse, immune system-rebuilding beneficial bacteria, and works wonders for the depressed immune system of the common American. Raw milk changes and saves lives, yet the FDA detests raw milk like nothing else on earth.

Pasteurization Killed Antibiotic Effectiveness for all of us: By creating a commodity dairy market system that relies heavily on antibiotics fed to heifers and dry cows at CAFO (Confined Animal Feeding Operation) the antibiotics now used in American hospitals for humans no longer work. Tens of thousands of Americans now die each year because of superbugs created by CAFO antibiotic abuse. MRSA and VRE (vancomycin resistant enterococcus drug resistance) are now a major cause of death, and there are fewer and sometimes no antibiotics left to kill the bad bugs and save human lives. The FDA refuses to ban or limit use of antibiotics in CAFO feed and instead testifies in defense of antibiotic use by the CAFO industry.

Pasteurization has killed the digestibility of milk and its delicious milk reputation. It triggers gas, allergies, diarrhea, asthma attacks, mucus production, constipation, gastric cramping and so-called "lactose intolerance." This has caused the dairy industry to lose many consumers to soy milk (suppresses thyroid function), rice milk, almond milk and even hemp milk. None of these fake milks comes from mammalian animals with teats.

The dairy industry time and time again claims that if you are black or if you are Asian you have a deficiency. You have something wrong with you. The fact of the matter is that the Masai in Africa and the Chinese outer Mongolians have drunk raw milk for thousands of years without lactose intolerance. There are virtually no human babies on earth that can't digest their own mothers' breast milk. That breast milk is raw milk. The same goes for nearly all grown or growing humans. The vast majority of people can drink raw milk if given a chance because the enzymes and lactase-producing bacteria that re-colonize the gut are found in raw milk. Raw milk is food for all people. It is color blind, unlike pasteurized milk produced by corporations seeking answers to the deficiencies found in their processed, dead partial milk. What people really are is "pasteurization intolerant." Fortunately, pasteurized milk has not killed the will of a small group of pioneering farmers and consumers to fight and expose the truth. This brings great news. Raw milk for humans is the solution and has exactly the opposite effect on farmers, the cows, the earth, the consumer—it is life-giving. Raw milk is now rapidly emerging as a farmer-to-consumer connected market. Things had to get really shockingly bad for the people and the farmers to see what really bad is.

Source for real food delivered to your door. **Clearview Valley Farm** www.clearviewvalleyfarm. com They offer Raw Milk and Dairy, Pastured Meats and more foods that are free of any chemicals, hormones, antibiotics, soy, and GMO's.

Nuts: one must purchase raw unpasteurized nuts and seeds. Nuts are highly nutritious. One ounce (28 grams) of mixed nuts contains:

- Calories: 173
- Protein: 5 grams
- Fat: 16 grams, including 9 grams of monounsaturated fat
- Carbs: 6 grams

- Fiber: 3 grams
- Vitamin E: 12% of the RDI
- Magnesium: 16% of the RDI
- Phosphorus: 13% of the RDI

Here are some of the most commonly consumed nuts:

- Almonds
- Brazil nuts
- Cashews
- Hazelnuts
- Macadamia nuts
- Pecans
- Pine nuts
- Pistachios
- Walnuts

Raw Nuts Are Antioxidant Powerhouses.

Antioxidants, including the polyphenols in nuts, can combat oxidative stress by neutralizing free radicals — unstable molecules that may cause cell damage and increase disease risk. The essential oils in nuts may protect your cells and lower' the LDL cholesterol preventing damage caused by free radicals.

One study found that walnuts have a greater capacity than fish to fight free radicals. Research shows that the antioxidants in walnuts and almonds can protect the delicate fats in your cells from being damaged by oxidation.

Raw Seeds: are an ancient food with a long list of potential health benefits that continues to grow. They're full of healthy fats and important vitamins, minerals and antioxidants. Some seeds are a great natural fast food to grab on-the-go, while other seeds are best added to salads, side dishes and recipes of all kinds.

Raw Flax Seeds

Compared to all other seeds and nuts, flaxseeds are an excellent source of fiber and the richest source of the omega-3 fat ALA (alpha-linolenic acid). Because the body doesn't easily digest the whole seed, it's best to eat ground flaxseeds so you're sure to absorb all the valuable nutrients. In several studies flaxseeds have helped lower cholesterol, blood pressure, and other risk factors for heart disease.

Ground flaxseeds can be easily mixed into non-dairy yogurt, smoothies, baked goods and chili or casseroles.

Warning: *Flax seeds have three times the amount of phytoestrogens than soy. For patients who have **cancer issues**, it behooves them to stay away from consuming these seeds.*

Raw **Chia Seeds**

Chia seeds are the tiniest of seeds and are a member of the mint family. Every 2 tablespoons pack 10 grams of fiber! That's 30-40% of the recommended fiber most people need for the day. For people with diabetes or pre-diabetes, chia seeds may help lower post-meal blood sugar (cinnamon has the same effect) because of this high fiber content. Just like flax seeds, chia seeds are an excellent source of ALA, but also calcium, magnesium and phosphorus – 3 important nutrients for bone health.

Chia seeds don't need to be ground like flax seeds and are also easy to add to your diet. Mix these tiny seeds with non-dairy yogurt, sprinkle on top of vegetables or soups, or try this Peach Chia Parfait.

For a delicious on-the-go snack with chia seeds, try Caveman Foods Grain-free Granola bars.

Raw Pumpkin Seeds

Pumpkin seeds are loaded with nutrition, including being one of the best natural sources of magnesium. Why is magnesium important? Most Americans don't get the recommended daily amount of magnesium and it's really important for:

- Controlling blood pressure
- Reducing heart disease risk

- Making & maintaining healthy bones
- Regulating blood sugar levels

People of all ages benefit from getting enough magnesium, so choose a handful of pumpkins seeds as a mid-afternoon snack.

Pumpkin seeds are also a good plant-based protein choice with 7 grams of protein in every ounce (¼ cup). Add ¼ cup to homemade trail mix or sprinkle on top of butternut squash soup, your favorite salad or other vegetable side dish to give it a protein boost.

Raw Sesame Seeds

These seeds haven't been studied as much as other seeds, but some research shows similar potential health benefits as other seeds, like lowering blood pressure and cholesterol and reducing inflammation. Sesame seeds can also help boost immunity because they have so many of the nutrients that play a key role in immunity (zinc, selenium, copper and iron). Keep in mind you need to eat at least 3 Tablespoons to get enough of a serving of these nutrients to make a difference. Like other seeds, they also have heart healthy fats, fiber and antioxidants.

Try adding sesame seeds to smoothies, hamburgers or meatloaf, and sprinkle a generous amount on stir-fry dishes and steamed vegetables.

Tip: Sesame seeds have vitamin T, which helps build platelets.

Raw Sunflower Seeds

Sunflower seeds are of special significance since they are high in omega 6 fatty acids. It is the omega 6 fatty acids that restore the integrity of your cell membranes. It is the omega 6 that acts as a magnet drawing oxygen into the cell. Of interest, **cancer cells cannot survive in a highly oxygenated environment.**

When you think sunflower seeds, think brain food. Omega 6 and omega 3 fatty acids present **Parent Essential Oils**. From these **Parent Essential Oils** the body makes DHA and EPA essential for brain function. They're also rich in three nutrients that have been shown to help protect the brain — vitamin E, magnesium and selenium. As a matter of fact, the brain uses more vitamin E than any other organ in the body. Just ¼ cup of these seeds gives you 2/3 of the recommended daily intake of vitamin E. Sunflower seeds also offer the same benefits of other seeds — reducing inflammation and risk of heart disease.

Sunflower seeds also provide a not-so-shabby 6 grams of plant-based protein in just 1/2 cup.

Add these seeds to burgers, tuna salad or chicken salad for a nutty crunch. Of course, they always make a great topping for salad or non-dairy yogurt. And for on-the-go snacks, eat a handful by itself or mixed with other trail mix ingredients, and many of our Caveman Foods bars have sunflower seeds as a key ingredient, including Nutrition bars, Grain-Free Granola bars and our new Grain-Free Granola Crunch!

With so many potential health benefits and so many seeds to choose from, it's time to make raw seeds a part of your daily eating routine.

Facts About Fats

In the past thirty years, fats have been linked to heart disease, clogged blood vessels, cancer, obesity and various degenerative diseases like arthritis, diabetes, cataract, multiple sclerosis, hypertension, nephritis, lupus erythematosus and others. As an attempt to combat these dreaded diseases, the medical profession and food industry, in recent years, have been promoting fat free products and avoidance of cholesterol rich foods. The real emphasis should be on avoiding all processed fats (hydrogenated, partially hydrogenated, and heated fats and oils), bleaching of flour and instead consume the only two essential fatty acids (linoleic acid [omega 6s] and alpha-linolenic acid [omega 3s]). The oils must be organic and cold pressed. Safflower and sunflower oils provide the omega 6s and chia seeds, brussels sprouts and avocado supply the omega 3s. The two essential oils provide the **Parent Essential Oils** from which the body can make all the other necessary oils.

The cholesterol scare has caused lay people and physicians alike to view all cholesterol as dangerous while driving some people almost to the point of being neurotic about eating foods high in cholesterol. Although eggs, butter, milk, cheese and fat meats are high in cholesterol they also carry the best antidote for it: phospholipids and lecithins. These phospholipids and associated factors of vitamin E protect the chromosome units in the cell. Without chromosome integrity, degenerative diseases occur.

The mantra of high cholesterol has also drummed up much business for the pharmaceutical industry who has profited enormously by the physician's compulsion to lower high cholesterol levels by means of statin drugs (they generate 29 billion dollars in worldwide sales). In the wake of misinformation and lack of proper nutrition, many people continue to suffer without resolution of their health problems.

Compounding the problem of a deficiency of ingesting good quality fats is the ubiquitous use of prescribed drugs in our society. The common use of aspirin to "Prevent" heart attacks and non-steroidal drugs to reduce inflammation, presents a major problem in that these drugs themselves block the normal metabolism of fats in the body. The fact remains that if patients are helped by the use of aspirin or non-steroidal drugs (NSAIDs), then one can infer that the patient has an underlying essential fatty acid (EFA) metabolism problem or deficiency. Correcting the EFA problem by means of high quality nutrition will not only improve the patients symptoms and decrease the need for medications, it will also help improve the patients overall health.

Fats are essential to bodily function. The EFA's enable saturated fats to be oxidized and provide heat and energy; they easily combine with protein and oxygen and pump them through the body; fats are also stored for body insulation and future utilization, used in cell membrane repair, secreted in milk and excreted in the feces. Fats are needed to replenish the fatty sheath around nerves, pad joints and organs and provide a vehicle for the fat soluble vitamins (D,E,K,A and F); they are also converted to other lipids which provide the basis for hormones and body fluids.

The essential fatty acids (EFA) are an integral fraction of fats important to the body. EFA's are unsaturated fats; they are unsaturated because they have bonds or linkages within their chemical structure which permit attachment of other essential compounds like protein and oxygen. When high quality, electron-rich fats are combined with proteins, the electrons are protected until needed by the body. The more bonds within the EFA structure the more beneficial the EFA is to the body. As an example, olive oil has only one unsaturated bond compared to flaxseed oil which has three. Another beneficial factor comes from the presence of a field of electrons when two or more bonds are present. These electrical charges are easily released within the body to recharge living substances, especially to the brain and nerves. It is this electrical property which is so vitally needed for enzyme reactions to sustain life. These essential fatty acids have favorable effects upon sex maturation, pregnancy, lactation and protect against the harmful action of x-ray irradiation. When deficient, the EFA's will increase bruising and strokes (capillary permeability) and high blood pressure (lower capillary resistance). They also are necessary in cholesterol metabolism and normal function of every cell and organ of the body. Strictly speaking the essential fatty acids (linolenic, arachidonic and linoleic) cannot be synthesized by the body and unfortunately most people's diets today are deficient in natural fats.

Natural fats fall into one of three families of fats. Each of these fats are converted into special hormones called prostaglandins (PGs). These prostaglandins act as chemical messengers within all cells and are essential to their normal function. Our bodies need all three types of EFA's in balanced amounts to provide the three types of prostaglandins (PG-1, PG-2 and PG-3). The PG-1's and PG-3's promote health and are considered beneficial to body function. These two groups decrease the clotting of blood, decrease blood pressure, decrease swelling, pain, and inflammation, **decrease tumor growth** and help burn fat. The PG-2 group does exactly the opposite and its functions promote the degenerative process.

The availability of the specific essential fatty acids from each of the families of fats is dependent on the fats not being processed (heated, partially or fully hydrogenated). The first family of fats (this group produces PG-1's) is comprised of those which are derived from food oils: safflower, corn, sunflower, peanut, evening primrose and black currant. The second group of fats (this group produces PG-2's) come from ingestion of red meats, dairy products, mollusks and shellfish. The last group of fats represent the cold weather oils: flaxseed (linseed), walnut, canola and from cold water fishes.

The biggest nutritional problem in our society today is the over consumption of processed fats. Most people are unaware of the quantity of processed fats consumed on a daily basis. Interestingly, when animals are fed solidified or saturated fats, they eat six times as much fat and six times as much food as compared to animals fed healthy unsaturated fats. When food labels are read, partially hydrogenated fats are in everything: margarine, all commercial peanut butters, most crackers, chips, cookies, cakes and candies, many breads, some mayonnaise and salad dressings as well as many of the commonly consumed foods. Processing natural fats to partially hydrogenated ones extend the shelf life of the product. The problem is that these partially hydrogenated fats interfere with the normal conversion of the group 1 and 3 fats to their appropriate prostaglandins. The end result of this faulty metabolism is the over production of PG-2 type which promotes inflammation, pain and degenerative diseases.

Health Benefits of Flaxseed Oil

Warning: cancer patients must minimize flax oil in their diet because they have three times the amount of phytoestrogens than soy! Phytoestrogens enhance the growth of cancer!

Excerpts from Healing Fats…Killing Fats by Udo Erasmus.

Richest source of omega-3 fatty acids (50-60% Omega-3s); contains almost twice as much of the mega-3s as fish oil.

Heart Disease — Omega-3s lower high blood cholesterol and triglyceride levels by as much as 25% and 65% respectively. Omega-3s decrease the probability of a clot blocking the artery in the brain (stroke), heart (heart attack), lungs (pulmonary embolism) or the organ (peripheral vascular disease…that is gangrene). Omega-3s will lower high blood pressure.

Cancers — Omega-3s dissolve tumors. Max Gerson used flax oil for this purpose in his clinic. Dr. Budwig in Germany has over 1000 documented cases of successful cancer treatment using flax oil along with additional support. She has been using flax oil successfully in cancer therapy for over 30 years now. More recent research shows that omega-3s kill human cancer cells on the same culture. Breast, lung and prostrate cancer cell lines were studied. Also note that organic omega 6 oils repair cell membranes and act as a magnet pulling oxygen into the cells. Cancers cannot survive in a highly oxygenated environment.

Diabetes — This disease, according to Dr. Budwig, has its origin in deficiency of omega-3s (as well as omega-6) fatty acids and is made worse by current lack of vitamins and minerals. Cell membranes deficient in organic, cold pressed omega 6 oils prevent the uptake of insulin and glucose raising one's blood sugar.

Arthritis — Omega-3's have been found to be effective in the successful treatment and prevention of arthritis. Both fish oils (**DO NOT** use fish oils: they are rancid at room temperature) and flax oil have been used. More recently, research using combinations of the omega-3 and -6 fatty acids found that 60% of rheumatoid arthritics were able to completely discontinue their non-steroidal anti-inflammatory drugs (NSAIDS) and another 20% were able to reduce their dosages of NSAID in half.

Asthma — Flax oil can relieve asthma noticeably, sometimes within a few days of starting to take the oil.

Premenstrual Syndrome — Many cases of PMS are completely relieved within one month with fresh flax oil. Vitamins and minerals are also very important.

Allergies — Omega-3s help to decrease allergic response. Since the body must be rebuilt, a longer time is needed before allergies are alleviated. Total nutritional support is required.

Inflammatory Tissue Conditions — Included here are the diseases which end in -itis, in which are meningitis, bursitis, tendinitis, tonsillitis, gastritis, ileitis, colitis, arthritis, phlebitis, prostatitis, nephritis, splenitis, hepatitis, pancreatitis, otitis, etc. as well as psoriasis and lupus. All of these inflammatory conditions may be helped by the Omega-3s.

Water Retention — Flax oil helps the kidneys remove sodium and water. Water retention (edema) is involved in swollen ankles, some forms of overweight, PMS, and late stages of cancer and cardiovascular disease.

Skin Conditions — Omega 6 oils (sunflower, safflower, walnut) is famous for its ability to make the skin smooth, soft and velvety. It will also alleviate those skin conditions whose origin is the lack of the omega-6s in the diet.

Vitality — One of the most noticeable signs of improved health from the use of flax oil is increased vitality, more energy. Athletes notice that their fatigued muscles recover from exercise more quickly. Omega-3s increase stamina.

Calmness Under Stress — Many people find this calming effect of fresh flax oil to be its most pleasant. Omega-3s fatty acids prevent excess toxic biochemicals which our bodies produce under stress.

Other Conditions — Flax oil can also be helpful in multiple sclerosis (in places where essential fatty acid consumption is high, multiple sclerosis is very rare); omega-3s are necessary for visual function (retina), adrenal function (stress), and sperm formation; cystic fibrosis (omega-3-containing oils will loosen the viscous mucous secretions and relieve breathing difficulties); some cases of sterility and miscarriage; some glandular malfunctions; some behavioral problems (schizophrenia, depression, manic-depressive disorder, etc.); addictions (to drugs or alcohol); and pathologically deviant behaviors.

Because they are the essential nutrients most commonly lacking in the North American diet, omega-3s are recommended for everybody. In order for the omega-3 fatty acids in flax oil to unfold their vital functions, the other essential nutrients (proteins, vitamins and minerals) must also be present in adequate amounts.

Carbohydrate Fiasco

Fructose: The Biggest Carb Culprit

People on low-carb diets lose weight in part because they get less fructose, a type of sugar that can be made into body fat quickly. Although fructose is naturally found in high levels in fruit, it is also added to many processed foods, especially in the form of high-fructose corn syrup. If your only source of fructose came from eating an apple or orange a day, keeping your total grams of fructose to below 25 per day, then it would not be an issue. *Cancer patients MUST totally avoid high fructose corn syrup!*

But what many completely fail to appreciate is that fructose is the NUMBER ONE source of calories in the United States and the typical person is consuming 75 grams of fructose each and every day. Because fructose is so cheap it is used in virtually all processed foods. The average person is consuming one-third of a pound of sugar every day, which is five ounces or 150 grams, half of which is fructose. This is 300 percent more than the amount that will trigger biochemical havoc, and this is the average — many consume more than twice that amount.

Evidence is mounting that excess sugar, and fructose in particular, is the primary factor in the obesity epidemic, so it's definitely a food you want to avoid if you want to lose weight. *For those people who were diagnosed with cancer, sugar feeds cancer cells and will speed up your demise.*

These "Healthful" Carbs Should be Avoided Too
By Joseph Mercola

Many dieters snack on pretzels in lieu of potato chips and other salty snacks, believing them to be healthier alternatives. But eating pretzels is akin to dipping a spoon straight into a bowl of sugar, as that's precisely the way your body responds to this refined carbohydrate snack.

Don't be fooled by the fact that they're "fat-free" — remember it's the carbs that are the culprit.

Your body prefers the carbohydrates in vegetables rather than grains because they slow the conversion to simple sugars like glucose, and decreases your insulin level. Remember when your insulin level rises, so does the inflammation through out your entire body. With increased inflammation comes fibrosis. Increased fibrosis causes blood vessels to clog, organs, especially your brain, to become fibrotic. Grain carbohydrates, like those in pretzels, will increase your insulin resistance (corrupted cell membranes due to adulterated omega 6 oils) and interfere with your ability to burn fat -- which is the last thing you want if you're trying to lose weight.

Even cereals, whether high-fiber, whole-grain or not, are not a food you want to eat if you're concerned about your weight. If they contain sugar, that will tend to increase your insulin levels even more … but even "healthy" sugarless cereals are an oxymoron, since grains rapidly break down to sugar in your body, stimulating insulin production and encouraging weight gain.

Of course, increasing numbers of people are now aware that refined carbs like white sugar and white bread may make them pack on the pounds. But many are still being misled that "good" carbs like whole grains and fruit won't. Remember, whether it's a whole grain, a sprouted grain or a refined grain, **ALL grains** rapidly break down to sugar, which causes your insulin resistance to increase and will make your weight problems worse and more importantly **feed cancer cells**! Insulin resistance can also result from adulterated fats, corn, soy, canola, cotton seed, sunflower, and safflower oils. These adulterated oils corrupt the cell membrane and reduce its permeability to insulin and cause your blood sugar to rise. It's called diabetes.

This is NOT the case with vegetables, however. Vegetables will NOT convert into sugar the way grains do, and most Americans need to eat far more vegetables. Eating carbs in the form of vegetables may make your carb intake higher, but will not be a hindrance to your health goals. One caveat, corn and potatoes do not count as vegetables; they act much more like grains as far as your body is concerned.

Digestive Enzymes vs Systemic Enzymes

Even though both are enzymes they have different functions. Digestive enzymes are present in raw foods. When raw foods are eaten, the digestive enzymes help breakdown the protein, carbohydrates, and fats that are present in the food. In a perfect world, we wouldn't need to take digestive enzymes if we ate raw foods directly taken from our garden. The problem is when raw food is shipped from California, Florida, or South America the living enzymes deteriorate. Within thirty seconds of cooking most of the enzymes are destroyed. For this reason it is essential that we take food based digestive enzymes to assist our body in breakdown the food components for absorption in our intestines.

Deficiencies in digestive enzymes are associated with a variety of health conditions, especially those that affect the pancreas as it secretes several key enzymes. Often these can be addressed with dietary changes, such as restricting certain foods or adding those with naturally occurring digestive enzymes, or by taking prescription or over-the-counter (OTC) enzyme supplements.

Digestive enzymes are substances secreted by the salivary glands and cells lining the stomach, pancreas, and small intestine to aid in the digestion of food. They do this by splitting the large, complex molecules that make up proteins, carbohydrates, and fats (macronutrients) into smaller ones, allowing the nutrients from these foods to be easily absorbed into the bloodstream and carried throughout the body.

Digestive enzymes are released both in anticipation of eating, when we first smell and taste food, as well as throughout the digestive process.

Each of the many different digestive enzymes targets a specific nutrient, splitting it up into a form that can eventually be absorbed. The most significant digestive enzymes are:

Amylase
Amylase is essential for the digestion of carbohydrates. It breaks down starches into sugars. Amylase is secreted by both the salivary glands and pancreas. The measurement of amylase levels in the blood is sometimes used as an aid in diagnosing various pancreas or other digestive tract diseases.

High levels of amylase in the blood may indicate a blocked or injured duct of the pancreas, pancreatic cancer, or acute pancreatitis, a sudden inflammation of the pancreas. Low levels may indicate chronic pancreatitis (on going inflammation of the pancreas) or liver disease.

Maltase
Maltase is secreted by the small intestine and is responsible for breaking down maltose (malt sugar) into glucose (simple sugar) that the body uses for energy. During digestion starch is partially transformed into maltose by amylases. The maltase then converts maltose into glucose that is either used immediately by the body or stored in the liver as glycogen for future use.

Lactase

Lactase (also called lactase-phlorizin hydrolase) is a type of enzyme that breaks down lactose, a sugar found in dairy products, into the simple sugars glucose and galactose. Lactase is produced by cells known as enterocytes that line the intestinal tract. Lactose that is not absorbed undergoes fermentation by bacteria and can result in gas and intestinal upset.

Lipase

Lipase is responsible for the breakdown of fats into fatty acids and glycerol (simple sugar alcohol). It's produced in small amounts by your mouth and stomach, and in larger amounts by your pancreas.

Proteases

Also called peptidases, proteolytic enzymes, or proteinases, these digestive enzymes break down proteins into amino acids. In addition, they play a role in numerous body processes, including cell division, blood clotting, and immune function.

Proteases are produced in the stomach and pancreas. The main ones are:

- **Pepsin:** Secreted by the stomach to break down proteins into peptides, or smaller groupings of amino acids, that are either absorbed or broken down further in the small intestine
- **Trypsin:** Forms when an enzyme secreted by the pancreas is activated by an enzyme in the small intestine. Trypsin then activates additional pancreatic enzymes, such as carboxypeptidase and chymotrypsin, to assist in breaking down peptides.
- **Chymotrypsin:** Breaks down peptides into free amino acids that can be absorbed by the intestinal wall. ***This enzyme is also effective against cancer cells.***
- **Carboxypeptidase A:** Secreted by the pancreas to split peptides into individual amino acids
- **Carboxypeptidase B:** Secreted by the pancreas, it breaks down basic amino acids.
- **Sucrase:** is secreted by the small intestine where it breaks down sucrose into fructose and glucose, simpler sugars that the body can absorb. Sucrase is found along the intestinal villi, tiny hair-like projections that line the intestine and shuttle nutrients into the bloodstream.

Digestive enzymes can be obtained from capsules or tablets which have concentrated digestive enzymes of various ratios of the different vegetable based enzymes. The other source is from raw foods. The following table provides the foods and their enzymes.

Foods with Digestive Enzymes		
Pineapple	Proteases (bromelain)	Helps digest proteins and has additional anti-inflammatory effects
Papaya	Proteases (papain)	Helps digest proteins and is a popular meat tenderizer
Kiwi	Proteases (actinidain)	In addition to its digestive enzymes, the fruit is high in fiber to support digestive processes and motility
Mango	Amylases	Helps break down carbohydrates from starches into simple sugars and increases as the fruit ripens
Banana	Amylases, glucosidases	Like amylases, glucosidases also break down complex carbohydrates
Raw honey	Amylases, Diastases, invertases, proteases	The amylases and diastases help to break down starches, invertases break down sugars, and proteases break down protein
Avocado	Lipases	Helps digest and metabolize fat
Kefir	Lipases, lactase, proteases	The lactase in kefir helps to digest the fermented milk and may be tolerated by some people with lactose intolerance
Saurkraut, kimchi	Lipases, proteases	Fermented foods develop enzymes during the fermentation process as well as probiotics, or beneficial bacteria, to further support digestive health
Miso	Lactases, lipases, proteases, amylases	This fermented soy paste contains a potent combination of enzymes that help break down lactose in dairy, fats, proteins, and carbohydrates
Ginger	Protease (zingibain)	In addition to its enzymes that can help break down proteins, ginger may also help ease nausea

The New Breed of Systemic Enzyme Blends by: Dr. William Wong ND, PhD

"Systemic enzymes are the most important part of maintaining a healthy body; of fighting the processes of both aging and disease; and of undoing the planned obsolescence nature has built into our bodies to make sure we don't stay on the planet for too long.

Systemic enzymes are the only non-toxic way of controlling inflammation of every type and from whatever reason. More importantly, systemic enzymes are the only tools available in both natural and allopathic (conventional) medicine for fighting fibrosis. We have to remember that most all disease names end with one of two suffixes, either the "itis" denoting an inflammation or an "osis" denoting a fibrosis condition. Most of what winds up killing man is either an inflammation (itis), such as heart and vascular disease, diabetes, cancer, trauma, Alzheimer's or a fibrosis (osis) related event such as a clot caused stroke or heart attack; fibrosis of the kidney, liver or heart valves; age related shrinking of the internal organs; etc. We also have to remember that of the two things that cause fibrosis, inflammation is the #1 major thing that brings about the formation of fibrosis and scar tissue. So control the one and you prevent the further formation of the other."

During these last 10 years, we have applied systemic enzymes to everything from simple osteoarthritis to auto immune conditions like RA and MS. In fibrosis conditions they were applied by docs for post-operative scar tissue to Glomerulosclerosis of the kidney and to Pulmonary Fibrosis in the lungs. Plastic surgeons were even preventing the formation of scar tissue and keloids on their work! With increase publicity more physicians and the public have become more aware and better able to understand the physiology and uses of proteolytic enzymes and the "new school" blends of systemic enzymes began flourishing.

Systemic enzyme formulas come in two-forms: vegetable based and animal based. German medical research shows that animal based systemic enzyme blends stay in the body working for 24 to 36 hours. While Indian pharmaceutical research shows that the purely vegetable based enzyme blends stay active in the body only some 4 to 6 hours. Research by pharmacologists have shown that real animal pancreatin does indeed absorb better and work better than the pancreatin imitations from vegetable sources. Research has also shown that not all pancreatin is equal. Most products containing animal based pancreatin are dilutions from the full strength pancreatin which is 12 to 14 times more powerful. Pancreatin is diluted by cutting it with lactose (milk sugar) until the desired dilution is achieved. According to the US Pharmacopoeia (the US formulary for pharmaceutical grade products) 1X USP has the ability to:

- Digest 25 times its weight in carbohydrates
- Digest 25 times its weight in proteins
- Digest 9 1/2 times it weights in fats.

If 1 X USP pancreatin can do that, then 12 to 14X USP will do 12 to 14 times the work! The added advantage of using a non-diluted pancreatin aside from its strength is that there is no lactose in the product to cause stomach upset in those who are lactose intolerant nor will it interfere with the enzyme activity of the Amylase in the product.

Dr. William Wong worked with the late Dr. Karl Ransberger, an enzymologist, to formulate the most powerful systemic enzyme product commercially available. Dr. Wong's formulation, Zymessence, provides five major actions:

1. It is anti-inflammatory.
2. It dissolves fibrosis or scar tissue.
3. It breaks down foreign protein in the blood.
4. It is bactericidal (kills bacteria)
5. It is mildly anti-viral.

Author's note: Systemic enzymes especially Zymessence has the ability to dissolve the biofilm secreted by cancer cells to protect itself from the body's immune system.

These five attributes provide a powerful natural approach to resolving cancer and any other major degenerative disease. It is the only systemic enzyme that is doubly enteric coated so that stomach acids do not reduce its potency. The key in the health equation is to enhance the terrain. The condition of the terrain is what dictates whether cancer or any other disease process will start. The six phases of detoxification that I alluded to in the beginning of this article is the key to establishing a healthy terrain. Remember, the germ theory is obsolete. The viruses, bacteria, fungi are the result of a toxic terrain and **NOT** the cause of the disease.

Nutritional Myths
by Dr. Richard Murray

MYTH: Americans are the best fed people on earth.

FACT: U. S. citizens are over fed but malnourished. The standard American diet is nutrient poor and rich in calories.

Doctor C. Everett Koop, former U.S. Surgeon General, has established that over 2/3 of all degenerative deaths in the United States are directly related to diet. The US is number one in the world in the number of colon cancer rates and diverticulitis.

MYTH: B-Complex deficiencies cannot exist in the US because all flour products (bread, pastas, cereals, etc.) are enriched with B vitamins and micronutrients.

FACT: The plants are greatly depleted of vitamins and minerals because of continued use of synthetic fertilizers. In addition, the B vitamins are quickly destroyed by microwave cooking and heat produced during normal cooking.

MYTH: Diet cannot control high blood pressure.

FACT: In Japan, high blood pressure is even more common than in the United States. In 1959, researchers compared two northern Japanese villages (Japan Heart Journal. 3:313-24, 1962). Both villages had similar sodium intake but different blood pressures. The group with the lower blood pressure was found to consume much more potassium in their diet. (The K Factor – Reversing and Preventing high Blood Pressure Without Drugs by Richard D. Moore, M.D., Ph. D and George D. Webb, Ph.D.)

Vegetarian groups consistently have lower average blood pressures than matched control groups) Lancet 1:5-9 [1983]).

MYTH: Vitamins and minerals in our body are not affected by medications.

FACT: Medications have a direct affect on our nutritional levels. For example, use of aspirin as recommended by many physicians to help prevent heart attacks will triple the loss of vitamin C and K. Use of oral contraceptives causes the loss of Vitamin C, Folic acid, B-12 and Calcium. Use of steroids decreases the body's levels of calcium, zinc, protein, vitamin D and C. (Food, nutrition and Diet Therapy- A Textbook of Nutritional Care by Marie V. Krause, B.S., M.S., R.D. and L. Kathleen Mahan, M.S., R.D. publisher W.B. Saunders).

MYTH: Nutritional supplements have nothing to do with bladder incontinence.

FACT: Bladder incontinence is the result of a weak muscle (sphincter) that controls the the neck of the bladder. This valve is nothing more than a band of smooth muscle. Smooth muscle gets its tone from natural B-complex vitamins in the diet. One of the best sources for natural B-Complex vitamins is from Standard Process Labs.

MYTH: The body cannot tell the difference between natural and synthetic vitamins.

FACT: Doctor Casimir Funk, the discoverer of vitamins and the first scientist to concentrate vitamin B stated, "The synthetic product is less effective and more toxic." The synthetic form is neither a mirror image nor even the same compound as the natural form. It does not work in a physiologic way but functions as a drug.

CHAPTER 11

COMPREHENSIVE APPROACH TO REVERSING CANCER

*C*ancer Deconstructed provides the reader with science based information to formulate a plan of action. The following bullet points enable the reader to quickly focus on the most important components of reversing cancer. Once you internalize this information, the fear will dissipate.

Bullet points of the most important components to reversing cancer

- Cancer is **NOT** a disease.
- Killing the cancer with toxic chemotherapy, radiation, or surgery is **NOT** solving the problem. If anything these treatments will reduce your quality of life.
- Cancer is an adaptation to toxicity.
- There are primary factors that trigger off cancer: 1) Adulterated omega 6 oils corrupt the cell membranes turning them into plastic, preventing oxygen to enter the cell; 2) Carcinogens block the 380 nm wavelength which heals DNA; 3) toxins lower the cell membrane potential to +55 millivolts, which triggers off cell proliferation.
- All cancers are the same.
- The primary initiating factor of cancer is hypoxia (low oxygen).
- A toxic terrain sets the stage for cancer formation.
- Eliminate all refined sugar, white bread, and whole grain breads from your diet.
- Cell membranes become plastic from adulterated omega 6 oils in our diet.

- A corrupt cell membrane prevents oxygen and nutrients from entering and waste products from leaving the cell.
- Organic, cold pressed omega 6 oils (safflower, sunflower, walnut oils) repairs the cell membranes.
- Organic, cold pressed omega 6 oils act as a magnet pulling in oxygen into the cell.
- Cancer cannot survive in a highly oxygenated environment; this is why ozone therapy is so effective.
- Eleven additional factors that impede the cell from functioning normally:

  1. Carcinogens (mercury, glyphosate, benzene, asbestos, radon, formaldehyde, fluoride, alcohol, etc.) block a band of ultraviolet light, 380nm, from entering the cell preventing repair of the DNA.
  2. Root canal teeth: provide toxic chemicals like hydrogen sulfide, thioethers, and mercaptans to further corrupt the cell membrane. There are numerous bacteria and viruses that are associated with dead teeth, which drain and concentrate into organs, tissues and cells.
  3. Cavitations or infections in the jawbone spew out a steady stream of toxins.
  4. Reduce wi-fi and other EMF exposure because they create systemic inflammation; if you live in a condo or apartment where your neighbor's wi-fi is in your bedroom you have to surround your bed with a faraday cage that is a curtain made of cloth material with silver threads woven in it.
  5. Processed foods provide chemicals, are devoid of nutrients and have no biophotons, which are needed to repair the DNA and other cell structures.
  6. Vaccines are loaded with toxic adjuvants some of which are cancer producing.
  7. Chlorine, bromine, and fluoride are halogens that suppress thyroid function, which suppresses the immune system.
  8. Psychological, chemical, and structural distress lowers the immune system.
  9. Nutritional deficiencies hamper mitochondria and cellular energy production.
  10. Acid pH lowers the oxygen levels and lowers one's pain threshold.
  11. Stop taking any fish oils. They are **ALL** rancid at room temperature and deplete $CoQ_{10,}$ which reduces energy production. They also help spread cancer cells.

- Follow through with the six phases of detoxification and stay faithful with the supplement schedule.
- Microwave cooking destroys the energy in the food and creates free radicals.
- Must filter your whole house water to remove the chemicals. Vitasalus, Inc. http://www.equinox-products.com/
- Coffee enemas quickly detox the liver.
- Lifestyle changes to remove poor dietary eating, more regular exercise, negative attitude, and psychological distress. Meditate and hug a tree at least once a day.
- Test and remove infected root canal teeth. Also test post-surgical areas of the jaw where teeth were previously removed.
- Recommend wearing Tesla Lightwear glasses especially when working on the computer to block the blue spectrum of light.
- Consider removal of mercury fillings especially if mercury is present in the cancer.
- Have a qualified practitioner test for residual infections in the throat where tonsils were removed. It's a hidden factor that suppresses the thyroid.
- Make sure your vitamin D_3 level is between 70ng/ml and 100ng/ml.
- Stop taking any synthetic vitamin formulas; only food based supplements that are tested compatible with your energy pattern.
- Drink fresh green juices from organic vegetables at least three times a week.

  1. Two Granny Smith apples
  2. One stalk of celery
  3. Two stalks of kale
  4. One large stalk of collard greens
  5. One carrot
  6. Small piece of beet
  7. Hand full of cilantro

- Eat more raw foods, raw dairy, organic vegetables, grass fed beef (no steroids, antibiotics or growth hormones); sashimi (avoid tuna - high in mercury).
- Turn off wi-fi at night and go hard wired for internet connection.
- Place a diode on your cell phone to protect you from the EMFs.

- Obtain a comprehensive evaluation to determine the causative factors.
- Have a practitioner test the appropriate food based supplements to remove the initiators.
- Have a qualified practitioner test the hospital's pathology slides of your cancer to determine the causative factors.
- Do daily 10 minute ozone treatments via ear ensufflation to flood the body with oxygen. Take vitamin E, N-acetyl-cysteine, selenium and omega 6/omega 3 right before treatment.
- Do a parasite cleanse with Ivermectin orally (one cc per 100 pounds with a second dose two weeks later), food grade diatomaceous earth, or artemsia, worm wood, and cloves. Two doses of Ivermectin coupled with food grade diatomaceous earth for 90 days is the most effective treatment.
- Use far infrared saunas to detox heavy metals and other poisons.
- Do the things that you enjoy the most on a regular basis.
- Learn to say NO to people so you are in control of your life.
- Avoid unnecessary invasive x-rays, surgeries, biopsies (will spread cancer cells) whenever possible.
- Say no to any vaccinations.
- Replace conventional fluorescent lights with full spectrum bulbs. Do not use LED lighting in your home. They give off wi-fi signals.
- Stop watching the conventional news, which is primarily negative.
- Stop listening to negative people's advise about why you should do chemotherapy.
- Change your circle of friends especially if they have negative attitudes.

The above recommendations may seem over whelming but remember it was the abuses that brought on the cancer by corrupting your body's terrain.

Ngui Matrix - Qigong acupuncture

One of the key considerations in your approach to cancer treatment is to raise your energy level. One method that is not well known is the use of the Ngui Matrix System of acupuncture. Dr. Stangley Ngui is a 23 rd generation Qigong grand master who practices in Richmond

Hill, Ontario (165 East Beaver Creek Rd. Unit 24 - Phone. 905.597.5007). I have studied under Dr. Ngui's tutilage and spent several days in his clinic observing him. I spoke with cancer patients who he reversed with just his Ngui Matrix acupuncture. To the average person this may seem bizzar, but it is well documented that balancing the energies in the body increases biophotons. It is the biophotons that Dr. Fritz Albert Popp discovered in the 1970s that repairs the DNA. It's not far fetched once you understand the mechanisms of healing. It makes more sense to tweak the body's Chi than to burden it with toxic chemotherapy, drugs, radiation, and invasive surgeries. The slash and burn mentality is barbaric, obsolete and destructive and yet many people out of fear still buy into this philosophy.

It was the late Carl Sagan, American astrophysicist, cosmologist, author and science educator who said that the universe is made up of electrons, protons, neutrons, and morons. It still amazes me that even when you present people with documented facts that their heighten fear prevents them from making an intelligent decision. A perfect example was a close friend of mine, who developed lung cancer and she opted for conventional toxic chemotherapy even though I presented her with actual patient case studies of lung cancer that were reversed with natural methods. Interestingly, my friend's brother who years earlier was diagnosed with pancreatic cancer went to a top tier cancer hospital and opted for the best chemotherapy money could buy. The men and women in the white coats killed him in record time. Knowing this she still went for the same illusion and suffered the same fate. One of my best friend's father, who was a doctor, always said, "there are no drugs for dumbness."

Theraphi System

The history of the origin of the Theraphi System dates back to the 1960s when Antoine Prioré did his experiments in France. Many of the experiments and tests were done by prestigious members of the French Academy of Sciences. Robert Courrier, head of the Biology Section: and Secretaire Perpetuel, personally introduced Priore's astounding results to the French Academy.

In the 1960's and 1970's, in France, Antoine Prioré built and tested electromagnetic healing machines of startling effectiveness. In hundreds and hundreds of strictly controlled tests with laboratory animals, Prioré's machine cured a wide variety of the most difficult kinds of terminal, fatal diseases known today. Funded by 16 million dollars, Prioré's machines concretely demonstrated a nearly 100% cure of all kinds of terminal cancers and leukemias, in thousands of rigorous laboratory tests with animals. These results were shown to medical scientists as early as 1960. The irony of Antoine Prioré research was that the French universities would not accept his results.

The operation of the Prioré machine was seemingly incomprehensible. Many orthodox French scientists—some of them world renowned—were outraged at the success of such a machine, shrilling that science had nothing to do with "black boxes:." They loudly called upon the inventor to explain the mechanism utilized by his machine, but the inventor either wouldn't or couldn't explain the curative mechanism. Prioré certainly knew how to build the machine and make it work. It is debatable to this day whether anyone— Prioré included —actually understood its principle of operation. Neither the French Academy nor Antoine Prioré knew anything of phase conjugation at the time.

Note: One of Prioré's intermediate devices cured terminal cancers and leukemias in thousands of laboratory animals.

In fact, the entire Western World knew nothing of phase conjugation in the 1960's when Prioré was getting his finest results. At that time, only the Soviets knew of time-reversed waves. Certainly Prioré 's machine was impressive. Into a tube containing a plasma of mercury and neon gas, a pulsed 9.4 gigahertz wave modulated upon a carrier frequency of 17 megahertz was introduced. These waves were produced by radio emitters and magnetrons in the presence of a 1,000 gauss magnetic field. Experimental animals were exposed to this magnetic field during irradiation, and the mixture of waves (some 17 or so) coming from the plasma tube and modulating and riding the magnetic field passed through the animals' bodies.

Prioré's equipment was reversed engineered and down sized. Paul Harris an electronic genius and quantum physicist, Dan Winter collaborated on the development of the Theraphi System. This device uses a Tesla coil to produce 500,000 volts and scalar waves that act as a carrier for

18 healing frequencies. I have been using this technology since 2016 with incredible results. It all comes down to changing the morphogen field that surrounds the cell.

Based on Antoine Prioré's Research of the 1960's and 70's the following attributes of Scalar Energy have been formulated:

1. Scalar energy is a phase-conjugated, double-helix that can reprogram mutated DNA of cancer cells into normal cells. Prioré had an almost 100 percent cure rate for all types of cancer in animals and humans.

2. Scalar energy can disassemble viruses, bacteria, fungi, heavy metals, chemicals, vaccines plus any foreign material, which the body can easily dispose of via its macrophage system.

3. Scalar energy can piggy back frequencies imprinting them into fluids.

4. By its ability to imprint frequencies into fluid, scalar energy provides the mechanism for storing memory in the body. Since the body fluids makes up 70 percent of our body, it acts as the antenna for attracting ambient scalar energy from our surroundings to help restore health. Eating raw foods, which stores scalar energy produced by the sun in the form of biophotons, is another source for restoring health.

5. Scalar energy has the ability to make new cells and repair old ones or whatever tissue(s) in the body by stimulating stem cells. In reality, it can transmutate anything that it needs. Thomas Galen Hieronymus in the 1940's proved that transmutation is possible.

6. Each organ or tissue in the body possesses a unique scalar energy harmonic.

7. Broadcasting a reverse-phase angle scalar energy harmonic of a disease back into the body will negate the condition.

Tesla Lightwear Optics

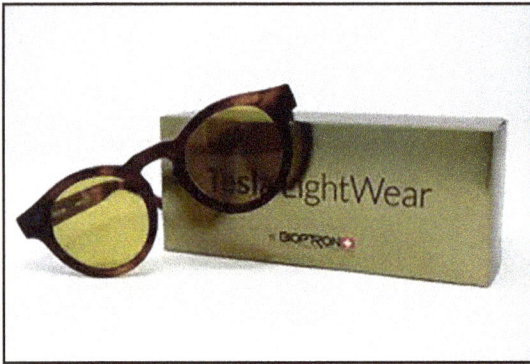

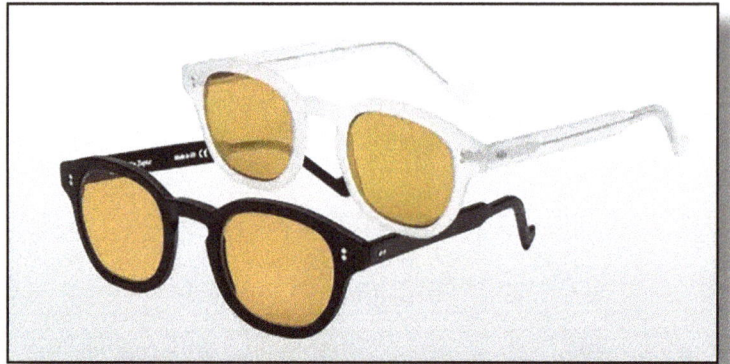

Light is the ultimate form of all electromagnetic energy. Light has dual wave-particle nature that has been revealed in quantum mechanics. This duality is shared by all primary constituents of nature. Through evolution, we became adapted to diffused sunlight, which includes high energy UV and a high-energy visible light (called blue-violet light from 380 to 450 nm) which keeps us on constant alert.

BIOPTRON has developed a method for transforming the light into a more beneficial form. Based on Zepter's patented technology and initial scientific pilot studies they recommend wearing the Tesla HyperLight Optics as a replacement for sunglasses, for blocking UV and highly energetic blue sunlight, as well as for possible relaxing effect, improved decision-making processes, and protection against the harmful portion of blue-violet light emitted by LCD and LED screens (as replacement for blue blocker glasses).

Today we spend more than 60% of our time in front of the computer screens and phone screens. When the artificial LED white light or LED from mobile devices and computers passes through the Tesla HyperLight Optics, it gets shifted into a light spectrum away from the harmful UV and blue-violet light and becomes hyperharmonized at the same time. The light spectrum of Tesla HyperLight Optics corresponds perfectly with the eye sensibility spectrum.

Quantum Healing with Hyperpolarized Sunglasses
by Gerald H. Smith, DDS, IMD

The use of light for healing is not a new concept. However, the use of hyperpolarized sunglasses as a new healing modality provides healthcare practitioners with an innovative technology that has great healing potential. The Swiss company, Zepter, has pioneered the use of man-made full-spectrum light for enhancing the body's ability to restore homeostasis. A recent clinical observation has spawned a new paradigm for patient treatment.

Since the human body functions within a normal frequency ranging from 62 to 68 MHz, any alteration that lowers the frequency range transitions the body into the disease state. It has been documented that disease starts at 58 MHz with the appearance of colds and flu at 57 to 60 MHz, Epstein-Barr virus occurs at 55 MHz, cancer initiates at 42 MHz, and death starts at 25 MHz. Elevating the body's frequency level by means of raw organic foods, homeopathic remedies, food based vitamins, minerals, scalar waves, essential oils, prayer and meditation, music, sunlight, Rife frequencies, and color light therapy all function to restore health.

Dr. Fritz Albert Popp discovered that carcinogens, like mercury, prevent the body from absorbing the wavelength of 380 nm to repair the DNA. This process triggers degeneration and disease. This blocking effect holds true for all carcinogens and prevents the DNA from repairing.

Fortuitously, this researcher recently discovered that placing the Tesla Lightwear glasses on someone who had a toxic substance like mercury in their pocket negates the deleterious effect of the mercury. The subject was tested kinesiologically to establish a baseline response. The muscles tested strong. Then a vial of mercury was placed in the subject's pocket, and the subject was retested. The retest resulted in the subject not being able to hold up their arms. The Tesla Lightwear glasses were then placed over the subject's eyes while the vial of mercury was still in their pocket, and the subject tested stronger than had been on the baseline test. My hypothesis is that the frequency generated by the vial of mercury disrupted the subject's energetic field. Placement of the Tesla Lightwear glasses stimulated the central and peripheral nervous systems, via the optic nerve, with full-spectrum light (430–770 THz

- minus the infrared and blue portions) to raise the energy field of the entire body from the inside outward. I believe this higher frequency has the beneficial effect of negating the 13 to 21 toxic frequencies that mercury produces. Extrapolating this finding, my theory is that wearing the Tesla Lightwear glasses will neutralize all toxic energy fields from pesticides, chemicals, heavy metals, vaccines, viruses, etc. by raising the frequency level of the body's energy field. In essence, the full-spectrum light will either transmutate toxic energy fields into nontoxic energy or erase them. Further study is needed to confirm these observations.

The Tesla Lightwear Sunglasses can be ordered directly from the North American division of Zepter International by calling (647) 748-1115.

The information presented in *Cancer Deconstructed* is based on innovative technology and clinical experience and represents knowledge that is at least fifty years ahead of mainstream medicine. My recommendation is do your own research. Do not take my word for it. Life is short; make the best of it and remember there are no luggage racks on hearses. God bless you.

APPENDIX A

ALKALIZING PROTOCOL

Steps – First thing in the morning and sequence throughout the day

- Always check first urine pH. An acid pH 5.0 denotes poor mineral reserves. Ideally 6.5 and above

1. Drink 1 glass of spring water (you may have to build up from 1/2 glass) + 1 wedge of organic grapefruit. To be given every hour. Give vitamins in #2 at same time.

2. Take one Potassium orotate and 4 magnesium orotate + 1/5 teaspoon of unpasturized raw honey. The Potassium and magnesium are only given in the morning. The raw honey acts as a carrier for the potassium and magnesium, which passes into the cancer cells along alkalizing and killing the cancer cells.

   Wait 10 to 15 minutes before doing next item.

3. Take 5 – 10 capsules of Proact Enz (digestive enzyme). Open and dump into 1/4 glass of spring water and add 1/2 teaspoonful of honey and one tablespoon of Aloe and blend in a blender to make a homogenized mixture. Give 4 times per day between meals. Designed to digest/breakdown the cancer cells.

   Wait one hour to complete next item.

4. Take Homozon* once a day in morning: Dissolve one teaspoonful of Homozon powder in 1/5th of a glass of water. In a second clean glass of water, squeeze

1/2 of a fresh organic lemon. Take immediately after patient drinks the Homozon. The citric acid from the lemon liberates oxygen from the Homozon powder.

5. Take one teaspoon of Coral Legend Powder and mix in 2 ounces of water. Give twice a day (11:00 am and before bedtime).

6. Between 4 O'clock and 6 O'clock but not later than 6 PM perform a coffee enema.

7. Take 1000 mg of AMLA -C (vitamin C) together with less than one ounce of water and 1/4 teaspoon of Pure Synergy powder. Take 2X per day but **not with enzymes.**

8. Take one Digest Enzyme with each meal.

This protocol is designed to alkalize the body, reduce fluid buildup and slow the growth of the cancer.

*   Homozon is available from ebay (https://www.ebay.com/itm/164299288090) $57 for 230 grams.

The Alkalizing Protocol is specifically designed to work like Insulin Potentiation Therapy (IPT) without the side effects of any chemotherapy drugs; IPT therapy gives the patient intravenous insulin to drop their blood sugar level; then a chemotherapy drug is given at one-tenth the normal dose. Cancer cells need sugar for their rapid proliferation. At one-tenth the normal dose the chemo drug does minimal collateral damage. Patients are also given raw sugar in the form of raw honey, which enables the chemo drug to get pulled into the cancer cells.

The above protocol achieves the same result but with natural substances. Also there is no adverse side effects since there is no chemotherapy drug given. This procedure is highly recommended especially in patients with advanced cancer. The ultimate objective is to restore the terrain of the body back to an alkaline oral pH of 7.5.

APPENDIX B

TESLA ENERGY CARD®

The Tesla Energy Card™ represents a new and innovative delivery system to balance the body's energy. The card has been programed with specific energy patterns to rebalance the body back to factory default. The frequencies also include a pattern that will activate the macrophage (like little Packman) cells to engulf foreign protein, viruses, bacteria, and chemicals that interfere with the body's immune system. In addition, it also has the frequency pattern of highly oxygenated water, which helps suppress cancer cells. It can also be worn 24/7 to help block Wi-Fi, EMFs and to effect a faster healing response. The card can be used repeatedly to imprint water bottles, food, and worn 24/7 for a period of six months from the date of first use. The card should be replaced due to diminished intensity of the energy pattern. It must be kept away from all cell phones, magnets, and electronic equipment to prevent erasure.

TESLA ENERGY CARD™
A New and Innovative Healing Delivery System

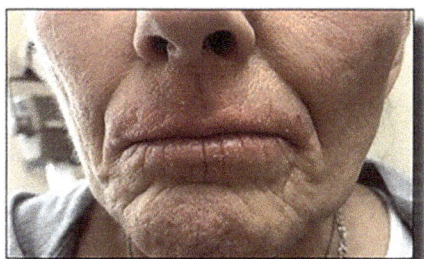

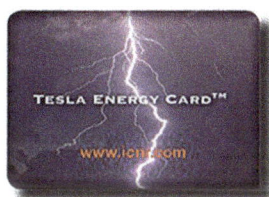

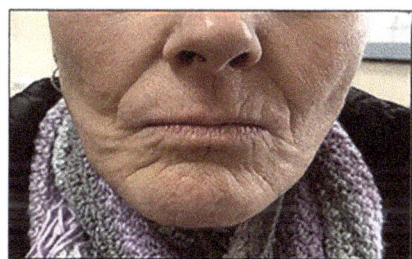

Before

24 Hours After

The patient was instructed to place a bottle of spring water that she normally drinks on top of the Tesla Energy Card™ and let it sit for five minutes before drinking. The magnetic strip on the Tesla Energy Card™ emits a proprietary blend of energies, which are imprinted into the water. Water acts like a crystal and can hold the energy pattern. By drinking the imprinted water, the energy enters the body and helps restore homeostasis. The patient stated, "I watched my lips go back to normal right before my eyes. I could not believe what I was seeing." The patient stated that she drank the water on Saturday, December 21, 2019 and by the next day Sunday, December 22, 2019 her mouth had been restored to normal.

"Better living through energy medicine"

APPENDIX C

VANISH PLUS: COUGHS, COLDS, AND FLU IMMUNE BOOSTER

Vanish Plus represents a new breed of delivery system that has evolved from decades of research and intelligent evolution. The clinically proven formula includes known immune boosters such as, 1,3 – 1,6 beta glucans, thymus (extract), food based vitamins A, C, E, vegetable based essential fatty acids, L-lysine, calcium lactate (non-dairy), zinc, cordyceps, and a proprietary blend of vibrationally charged immune boosters that activate the body's own defenses to engage pathogens (viruses, bacteria, mold, fungus, etc.). Vanish Plus comes in a convenient two-ounce spray bottle. Dosage: Six sprays orally taken three times a day away from foods allows the vibrationally infused liquid to be quickly absorbed into your bloodstream.

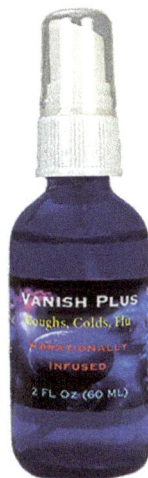

Available from www.teslaenergy-tec.com $19.95

OMEGA 369 PLUS: CBD ON STEROIDS

Omega 369 Plus has quadruple the effectiveness of conventional hemp derived oils; this was accomplished by vibrationally infusing it with frequencies of four different high quality energy patterns derived from original organic hemp sources. All four original base samples were organically farmed, non-GMO, with no psychoactive THC, and rich in frequencies derived from cannabinoids and terpenes for enhanced effect. Our original organic base hemp source had the highest energy levels of cannabinoids and terpenes content of any hemp farm in the US. Our proprietary formula, Omega 369 PLUS, complements the vibrational frequencies of four sources derived from hemp with additional healing frequencies to further enhance the immune system and reset the body back to factory default. Our carrier is made up of certified organic, cold pressed sunflower oil, pumpkin seed oil, extra virgin coconut oil, and caprylic acid derived from coconut to further enhance absorption and improve brain function. The vibrationally infused frequencies have the added advantage of penetrating cell membranes faster than any other product on the market.

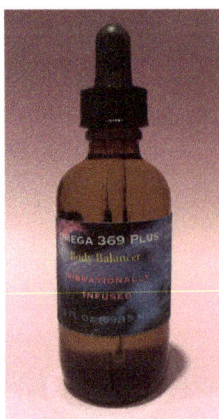

Available at www.teslaenergy-tec.com $125.00

APPENDIX E

KAQUN WATER

KAQUN water was born as a result of Dr. Robert Lyon's research work of twenty years. This drinking water is made with a special procedure - The Kaqun Technology™. The first device able to bind the active oxygen in pure water was made in 1981. After that, twenty years of research work and development followed when the high oxygen content KAQUN water could come into the consumer market.

KAQUN water is the only currently known water that has undergone 10+ years of clinical and laboratory research carried out on both healthy volunteers and those with health challenges, as well as animal studies (https://kaqun.eu/studies).

KAQUN water represents an absolutely unique development in water chemistry that is able to prevent hypoxia (the lack of oxygen in the body) without side-effects, due to its highly-bound oxygen content. Kaqun water is created by a specific treatment process that enables substantially increased absorption effects in the body. As a result of KAQUN technology, oxygen has been made into a stabilized form with concentrations of 18-25 mg per liter.

There are no chemicals or toxic materials used in the production of KAQUN, and the oxygen is derived from the water itself - not from an outside source.

There are two-forms in which KAQUN water is delivered to the body: through the skin (KAQUN baths) and by drinking a milder form of the KAQUN water (KAQUN drinking water). KAQUN has been shown to reduce mental and physical tiredness since it replenishes oxygen to the cellular environment within a short period of time. It will be quickly absorbed through the cell membrane even though it maybe corrupted with adulterated omega 6 oils from processed foods.

KAQUN water is not your typical mineral water. It possesses a low mineral concentration because it has undergone an initial purification process. By way of the hyper-oxygenation process of KAQUN, regular consumption has been shown to detoxify, refresh, energize, as well as enhancing athletic performance. By establishing a highly oxygenated environment, it has the potential of inhibiting the growth of cancer. Kaqun water is a must for anyone diagnosed with cancer.